PTERYGIUM SURGERY

LUCIO BURATTO, M.D.
ROBERT L. PHILLIPS, M.D.
GIUSEPPE CARITO, M.D.

MEDICAL ILLUSTRATIONS ZELDA ROCCHI

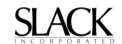
SLACK
INCORPORATED
6900 Grove Road • Thorofare, NJ • 08086

Publisher: John H Bond
Editorial Director: Amy E. Drummond

Pterygium surgery/[edited by] Lucio Buratto, Robert L. Phillips, Giuseppe Carito.
    p. ; cm
    Pterygium Surgery
    Includes bibliographical references.
    ISBN 1-55642-492-2 (alk. paper).

Printed in Italy by Litografia Fabiano - Milano

Published by: SLACK Incorporated
                6900 Grove Road
                Thorofare, NJ 08086-9447 USA
                Telephone: 856-848-1000
                Fax: 856-853-5991
                World Wide Web: http://www.slackbooks.com

Contact SLACK Incorporated for more information about other books in this field or about the availability of our books from distributors outside the United States.

Last digit is print number: 10 9 8 7 6 5 4 3 2 1

DEDICATION

To my brother Licinio
Who after many years of suffering has rediscovered
The joys of love and the joys of living.

Lucio Buratto, M.D.

———— ———— ———— ———— ————

To John W. Reed, M.D.- a friend, a teacher and an inspiration to all his fortunate colleagues.
John stimulated my life-long interest in cornea and external disease, and I will be forever in
his debt for the fund of knowledge that I have used throughout my professional career. John
has patiently imparted his knowledge to many over the years, and he remains the epitome of
an excellent and conscientious physician engaged in the ethical practice of medicine, and an
individual whom all can emulate with pride.

R.L. Phillips, M.D.

———— ———— ———— ———— ————

To my father with my deepest gratitude.

Giuseppe Carito, M.D.

CONTENTS

PART A

PART B

ACKNOWLEDGMENTS

During my life I have been extremely fortunate to have met many 'stars' of eye surgery.
One in particular stands out in my mind: a true surgeon, with depth knowledge of the subject,
a person wholly committed to the continual improvement in the field of corneal surgery.
His name is Giovanni Rama.
A special thanks to Dr. Marco Moncalvi.

Lucio Buratto, M.D.

There are often so many people to thank in a project as large as the publication of a book, and not enough space to adequately do so. Primarily I want to thank Michelle McKnight, C.M.T., whose considerable expertise and patience guided me through some uncharted waters, and from whom I appreciate very much the suggestions and help in many ways. Michelle is a credit to her profession, and without her help my contribution to this book would not be possible.
Brooke Williams, C.P.A., was always ready to help with a cheerful demeanor and considerable computer knowledge that helped us through the entire process. Brooke was never hesitant to stop what she was doing and lend a hand.
Vikki Kristiansson from SLACK was always readily available to give me some advice when I needed it, and also encouragement along the way, that this project could actually be completed if I would just keep working. John Bond and Amy Drummond from SLACK, with whom I had many early conversations regarding the concept of a book on pterygium surgery, both continued to encourage me to overcome my constant procrastination and take the first step.
And finally, I would like to express grateful appreciation to Lucio Buratto, whose vision and energy led to both the inception of the book and also its completion. Lucio continued to rouse me from my lethargy, set deadlines, and make me understand that we should not only be concerned with the quality of our work but also with the timeliness of its completion.
In closing, I would like to thank the many Residents who have rotated through the Cornea Service at the University of Alabama, both known and unknown, who have encouraged me in small and great ways to continue to try and refine techniques and methodology for pterygium surgery. Their insightful questions and comments would always lead to new ideas, and for that they all have my gratitude. My wife, Pam, my children, David, Michael, and Jennifer, have all been a source of encouragement and support through frustrating times, and ones that were not only concerned with the book but also maintaining a practice and all the other activities that go on in Departments of Ophthalmology.
To all of the above individuals, and some others that I have probably overlooked, you, too, have had a part in this publication, and for that I thank you all.

Robert L. Phillips, M.D.

CHAPTER CONTRIBUTING AUTHORS

Rafael I. Barraquer
Barcelona, Spain

Lucio Buratto
Milan, Italy

Giuseppe Carito
Venice, Italy

Robert Cionni
Cincinnati, Ohio

Joseph Frucht-Pery
Jerusalem, Israel

Robert L. Phillips
Birmingham, Alabama

Charalambos S. Siganos
Crete, Greece

Abraham Solomon
Miami, Florida

Donald T.H. Tan
Singapore, Singapore

Scheffer C.G. Tseng
Miami, Florida

Todd Watanabe
Cincinnati, Ohio

PREFACE

Over many centuries eye surgeons have struggled to perfect methodology to deal with the enigma of pterygia. From at least 1000 B.C. there are writings chronicling a variety of techniques employed to try and eliminate this seemingly simple growth. Yet to the present day, pterygia remain somewhat of an enigma, and there is no universal agreement as to the best treatment. While recurrence rates have decreased over many years, as new therapies have become available, there are pterygia for which the surgery does nothing more than stimulate aggressive behavior. This book, with a large number of contributors, will attempt to give the reader an overview and a more complete perspective of the many approaches available to this most perplexing disease.

There is no current unanimous opinion as to the best possible management for this pathology. This book reflects the fact that there is no universal agreement, and therein lies its strength. While we all agree on certain basic concepts, there are always variations of surgical and medical techniques employed to treat this disease, and this book reflects a diversity of opinion among many excellent surgeons. While these differences of opinion are not great, there are enough nuances of different thought that the reader can pick techniques and methodologies best suited for his or her particular level of skill.

The authors want this to be a "how-to" book that will be simple and concise, and try to provide readers with a fund of knowledge that can increase their confidence in their ability to handle both the simple and the complicated case. It is important that one be familiar with all the modalities of treatments, so that a proper choice can be made between the many approaches available, such as conjunctival flaps or grafts, lamellar keratoplasties, beta-irradiation, Argon laser, or the use of Mitomycin therapy.

Even though sometimes it might be tedious, it is important that we know where we have been in order to chart our path for the future. Historical theories of pathogenesis can still be relevant even today because it is important to know what did not work in order to gain some insight for the future. Different processes are probably at work in the recurrence of pterygia, and there may be individual variations in terms of climate, ultraviolet light exposure, and even variations from individual to individual down to the molecular level.

The work of all of us has been made more fruitful by the contributions of many authors around the world, and the bibliography in this book reflects the work of many individuals who have contributed important ideas.

Over the last several years, new information regarding the role of limbal stem cells and more recently, the use of amniotic membrane transplants have ushered in a whole new area, not only in surface correction in a wide variety of corneal problems, but also in severe pterygia recurrences. As more knowledge is gained in the use of the amniotic membrane grafts, Mitomycin and other modalities, our recurrence rates continue to decrease and our knowledge base continues to grow.

New modalities require continued training to become confident in their use, and caution is always required when applying new methodologies.

All pterygium surgeons are indebted to Kunitomo and Mori, who first reported the usefulness of postoperative instillation of Mitomycin to suppress fibroblastic activity. The pharmacokinetics of this medication are still under investigation, and more needs to be learned. We have learned to develop extreme caution with its use, and found that an intraoperative instillation may be all that is necessary, and will avoid the significant risk when used as a postoperative drop. A significant portion of this book is devoted to allow the reader to learn everything that is known regarding the action of Mitomycin, and also the reader is made aware of the extreme caution that must be exercised, and when the drug might be contraindicated. All of these issues must be carefully explained to the patient so that each individual is made well aware of the benefits of this drug and also the potential problems, which can be significant.

The authors have tried to outline in significant detail, a variety of surgical techniques that can be applied to this disease. Some of the descriptions of these techniques is very detailed. But, as in most surgical procedures, to gain complete authority in the exercise of a surgical methodology, it is important to be detailed and precise. The collective cases of the authors are very significant in number, and it is hoped that the reader can take advantage of the combined wisdom and experience of a number of people who have differing points of view. One learns about surgery not only from seeing the reported successes but also about learning from failures and complications, and those are illustrated in this text as well.

In closing, the desire of the co-authors and contributors has been to gather together as much expertise as possible that can be brought to bear on this subject, so that the reader will have a useful guide to both the historical past and the promise of the future. By design, the authors have included overlapping and repetitious information, as well as significant differences of opinion, to allow readers to choose the right perspectives for their own practices. Each pterygium surgeon must try to seek his own level of understanding and comfort, because not every procedure will be needed for every surgeon. This book allows individuals to pick and choose a variety and combination of techniques that will suit their own surgical practice, and hopefully from the 21 chapters will gain a better understanding of the very best possible way to approach both primary and recurrent disease, as well as complications of the treatments themselves. Pterygia surgery will never lend itself to complete agreement and unanimity of thought, and in differences of approach the strength of this book is made paramount. We all look forward with interest to future developments in the treatment of this disease.

Robert L. Phillips, M.D., F.A.C.S.
Associate Professor of Ophthalmology
University of Alabama
Birmingham, Alabama

PART A

LUCIO BURATTO, *M.D.*
GIUSEPPE CARITO, *M.D.*
ROBERT J. CIONNI, *M.D.*
ROBERT L. PHILLIPS, *M.D.*
TODD M. WATANABE, *M.D.*

1

INTRODUCTION

A pterygium is just one of the primitive degenerative and hyperplastic pathologies of the conjunctiva. It is different to other similar clinical forms the so-called pseudo-pterygium - through its etiology.

In its traditional definition, a pterygium is the appearance of a fibrovascular neo-formation which arises in the conjunctiva and grows towards and infiltrates the surface of the cornea. It is normally triangular in shape with the apex or head pointing towards the center of the cornea and the base facing the semilunar fold, at the medial canthus.

A pterygium evolves very slowly over the years from the limbus where it would appear to originate; the evolution is not constant as there are periods of clinical calm and so-called inflammatory episodes with more rapid growth. Generally speaking, the progression is extremely slow. In the progressive forms, the pterygium grows and extends towards the center of the cornea with a clinical behavior similar to neo-formations of the eye surface that is infiltration of the cornea, and a tendency to recur following removal. In the initial or stationary forms, the job of the eye surgeon is limited to the evaluation of the clinical picture and the control of the evolution.

Treatment is not indicated in these cases, but sometimes the patient himself will request the operation to remove the pterygium either for aesthetic reasons *(Figures 1-1 and 1-2)* or because it reduces the patient's tolerance levels to contact lenses. In the more advanced forms, when the pterygium has invaded the cornea, the evolution worries the patient. He will consult an eye surgeon because of the

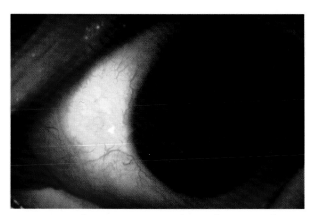

Figure 1-1. *Small primary pterygium. This small pterygium does not cause any irritation and the patient himself did not complain of any inflammatory episodes. The lesion did not show any signs of progression over the years. There are no indications for surgery.*

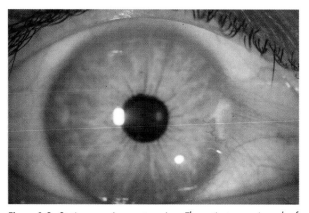

Figure 1-2. *Stationary primary pterygium. The patient, myopic and soft contact lens wearer, complained of reduction in tolerance to the contact lenses in the eye affected by pterygium, with uncomfortable irritation which requires surgical treatment. For this reason, despite the fact that there is no progression of the disease, treatment is indicated.*

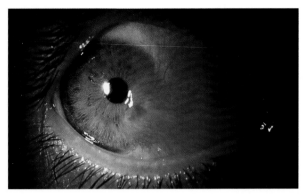

Figure 1-3. *Progressive primary pterygium. Because of his profession, the patient is subject to considerable exposure to environmental UV light. For the last two years, he has complained of inflammation with growth of pterygium. The photo shows a bout of inflammation with considerable congestion of the body and the head of the pterygium, the progression of which threatens to invade the optical zone. Surgery is indicated.*

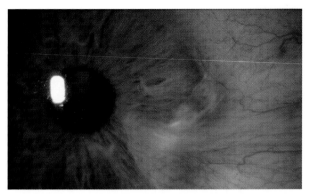

Figure 1-5. *Recurrent pterygium. In this patient operated on three years earlier, there are no clinical signs of progression and the disturbance is essentially due to a mild irregular astigmatism. The head invades the peripheral cornea and the surrounding opacity is close to the optical zone without invading it. The body of pterygium is clearly visible and extends as far as the medial canthus. Surgery in these cases is not indicated to avoid exposing the pterygium to further recurrence which may be even worse than the previous growth.*

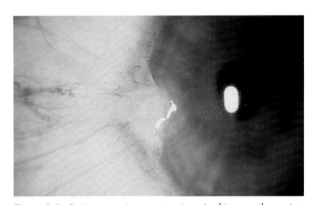

Figure 1-4. *Stationary primary pterygium. In this case the patient complained that the pterygium had not progressed over the previous years and there had been no prolonged episodes of redness but just an occasional sensation of foreign body due to contact between the eyelid and the head of the pterygium raised on the cornea. The indication for surgery in these cases must be considered with caution and is necessary only when the irritation increases or when there is inflammation with signs of new growth.*

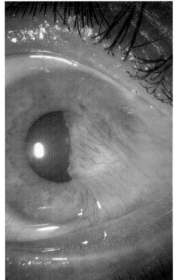

Figure 1-6. *Evolved primary pterygium. The patient is a 63-year-old fisherman who reported the appearance of pterygium at about 25 years of age. He reported numerous episodes of inflammation over the subsequent years with progressive growth of the lesion. Vision is greatly compromised because of the invasion of the optical zone. Over the last two years, the patient complains of uncomfortable diplopia in lateral gaze. The surgical treatment of these forms is always indicated; the surgeon must have considerable experience in the field of corneal surgery and conjunctival repair with mucosal grafts.*

worsening, or because of the appearance of irritation or because of a reduction in vision. In these cases, the surgeon must identify the indicators of clinical evolution and suggest the most suitable surgical treatment *(Figures 1-3, 1-4, 1-5)*.

In cases of a highly advanced pterygium, the growth on the cornea and the invasion of the pupil will always require surgery which must be performed by an experienced surgeon.

Under these circumstances, the eye surgeon is faced with some delicate problems such as the treatment of the optical zone *(Figures 1-6, 1-7)* the recurrences and the repair of the conjunctiva.

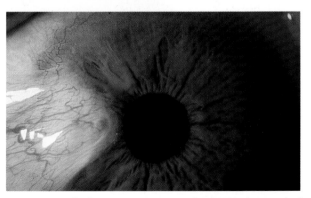

Figure 1-7. *Evolved primary pterygium. In this patient, the growth of the pterygium has marginally reached the optical zone causing a reduction in the vision with considerable disturbances in night vision. Surgery is indicated.*

2

HISTORICAL BACKGROUND

On examination of the scientific literature, we were astonished at the attention pterygia have been given over the thousands of years of Medical History.

The most famous doctors of ancient times were interested in pterygia, and, they gave the condition their own personal explanation and described with great precision the various clinical conditions. Pterygia were already distinct from other conditions with a similar appearance and the doctors at that time were already aware of its clinical importance and the frequent recurrences.

Susruta, for example, an Egyptian doctor who lived in 1000 bc. gave an accurate description of a pterygium and its treatment with pulverized salt and stimulation with a palm branch. When the pterygium was inflamed and swollen, he tore it out with forceps and removed any remaining tissue with a flesh-stripping ointment. He also described the ease with which the lesion reappeared.

Hippocrates (469 bc.) suggested the use of eye-drops containing lead, zinc, copper, iron, bile juices, urine and maternal milk.

Celso (50 ac.) and Galeno (131 ac.)[1,2] also suggested a topical treatment with solutions of white wine, vinegar, euphrasy water, candied sugar, nitrated fennel water and, in the more serious forms, the physical removal. This was done by passing a thread underneath the growth and allowing it to slide over the scleral surface with a to-and-fro movement as far as the medial canthus; then when the pterygium was detached from the underlying sclera, it was cut with scissors.

Other indications were given by Paolo Egineta (660 ac.) and the Arab Avicenna (1037 ac.) who suggested cutting the pterygium with scissors.

Ambrose Pare (XVI century) wrote about a pterygium: "You have learned that a pterygium is an illness that always recurs, even when you have done everything in your power to cure it"; this concept has remained true to the present day.

In the XVIII century, it was fashionable to treat a pterygium with copper sulfate, in the XIX century with silver nitrate and lead acetate, and atropine was added to encourage the healing of the associated corneal ulcers.

The XIX century saw the advent of surgery of pterygia:

- **Scarpa** (1802): removal of the head from the cornea using forceps, section of a portion of the body (3-4 mm) and subsequent concentric excision of the detached tissue as far as the limbus.[3]

- **Arlt** (1850): excision of the head from the cornea and a diamond-shaped portion of the body with conjunctival cross-over plastic surgery.

- **Desmarres** (1855): introduces the technique of deviating the head in an attempt to change the direction of growth and induce it to atrophy.[4] The technique was modified by Terrien[5] who deviated the growth towards the superior fornix as opposed to the inferior fornix suggested by Desmarres.

- **Knapp** (1869): suggested the technique of transposition. The pterygium is cut longitudinally into two halves that are fixed below the superior and inferior conjunctiva.

- **Arlt** (1872): he performed the first scleral repair following the excision of the pterygium with the addition of autologous or homologous cadaver conjunctiva.
- **Klein** (1876): performed Arlt's technique but he used mucous tissue from other sites.

In the XX century, thanks to progress in the field of medical physics and biotechnology, the techniques of keratoplasty and the physical treatments of pterygium were developed.

In the Twentieth century, we can mention:

- **McReynolds** (1902) who presented a modified Desmarres technique which placed the head of the pterygium in a conjunctival pouch.
- **Gifford** (1909) used a thin epidermal graft to cover the sclera that was exposed following the complete removal of the pterygium.
- **Morax** and **Magitot** (1911) used the first artificially-preserved homologous corneal grafts.
- **Terson** (1911) was the first to use radiation therapy with X-rays.
- **Fuchs** (1911) presented the first results of autologous penetrating keratoplasty for the treatment of corneal pathologies, and Terson (1913) performed this on pterygia. The technique involved replacing a full-depth corneal disc containing the head of the pterygium with a penetrating disc of the same diameter removed from the superior peripheral cornea. The results were poor because of an opacity which developed in both discs, and because of an inaccurate surgical technique and because of trophism and infection. The author also reported cases of eyes lost through postoperative infection.

Until then the research had examined the conjunctival component alone, so for the first time, the problem of the corneal treatment of pterygium was brought into focus.

- **Magitot** (1916) suggested lamellar autokeratoplasty using a technique which is similar to Terson's but which used lamellar disks removed from the same eye.
- **Elschnig** (1926): in order to repair serious conjunctival defects, he performed conjunctival plastic surgery with transposition of a bridge created from the contro-lateral limbus.
- **Amorin** (1936) suggested treatment with a diathermy coagulator.
- **Burnam** and **Neil** (1941) used a radioactive applicator (Radon)
- **Kamel** (1946) performed sub-conjunctival cauterization of the pterygium with carbolic acid.
- **D'Ombrain** (1948) suggested the technique of scleral baring for the first time.
- **Paufique** (1950s) developed a lamellar keratoplasty for the optic and therapeutic treatment of the corneal pathologies; this also included the pterygium which until then considered to be a minor pathology.
- **Haik** (1957) used topical beta-therapy with strontium 90 (Sr90)
- **Meacham** (1962) was the first to use antimitotics to prevent the recurrences.
- **Panzardi** (1964) used amniotic membrane to repair the conjunctival tissue loss following excision of the pterygium.
- **Kenyon** (1985) reported excellent results in the prevention of recurrences by grafting autologous conjunctiva to the limbus.

3

EPIDEMIOLOGY

A pterygium is more common in warm sunny geographical areas; elsewhere the prevalence is low or negligible. In the temperate regions, the prevalence in the population lies at about 2% whereas in tropical regions, it reaches a prevalence ranging between a minimum of 6% to more than 20%.[9,111]

Pterygia are most common in the tropics in an equatorial zone between the 30th Northern and Southern parallels. When we leave this zone, the prevalence in the population is progressively reduced.

- A low percentage, between 0% and 1.9% is reported beyond the 40th parallel (Scandinavia, Germany, Russia, United Kingdom, the north of France, Canada and the northern states of USA).

- A moderate percentage, between 2% and 4.9%, is observed between the 35th and the 40th parallels (South of Spain, South of Italy, North Africa, the central regions of USA).

- A high percentage, between 5% and 10%, is observed between the 30th and 35th parallels (the southern states of USA, Egypt and China).

- A very high percentage, more than 10%, in the regions between the 30th parallel and the equator (Australia, India, Pakistan, equatorial Africa and Central America). In some of the aborigine tribes in Australia, the prevalence can reach 90%.

Epidemiological studies on populations of vast geographical areas have highlighted the role played by the environmental factors on the pathogenesis of pterygium, with the identification of the major and minor risk factors.

The correlation with the exposure to UV sunlight is evident and universally accepted. Pterygia may develop when exposure is a daily event, and prolonged for years.

Young adults in their twenties run a greater risk of being affected by environmental UV light.[12,22,14,15,18]

Ultraviolet light (UV) is also associated with other hyperplastic/degenerative pathologies and tumors of the eye surface and the skin.[11,13,14,18]

Obviously certain groups of people are more exposed to the risk: farmers, sailors and fishermen, builders, welders and any one else who spends a lot of time outdoors exposed to sunlight. Taylor reported that the environmental and climatic factors have a greater influence in geographical areas where the mean annual relative humidity lies between 40% and 59%, as opposed to sandy areas where there is a dry, ventilated climate.[12,13,22,51]

There is a slightly greater prevalence of pterygia in male subjects and the mean age for onset is 44 years, with a peak in the a patients aged between 50-60 years.[10,112]

Some races have a greater predisposition to pterygia, for example, Indians are affected more

PREVALENCE OF PTERYGIUM IN THE WORLD (Cameron)	
Latitude (parallel)	prevalence
Beyond 40°	0% - 1.9%
35°-40°	2% - 4.9%
30°-35°	5% - 10%
30° - equator	more than 10%

than Caucasians, Thais more than Chinese, dark-skinned Africans more than pale-skinned Arabs.

RISK FACTORS

The main or primary risk factors in the onset of pterygia can be identified in the life-style and profession of the patient and it is the ophthalmologist's job to be aware of this and inform the patient on the role these play in the clinical evolution of the lesion.

The patient exposed to greatest risk is the young adult, who for professional or environmental reasons, is subject to daily exposure to UV radiation, particularly if he does not use sunglasses or protective shades.

According to some authors, pterygia are transmitted with pluri-hereditary factors with incomplete penetration and variable expression.[8,113,114]

Duke-Elder reported dominant heredity with low penetration, but this did not refer to the lesion itself but to a predisposition of the conjunctiva reacting abnormally to the atmospheric/environmental stimuli.[10,17,18]

It has been observed that in some families the incidence of pterygia is much higher than the geographical average suggesting that a hereditary factor is likely.

However, it is still unclear whether it is a genetic issue or whether the family and its components are exposed to the same risk factors for several generations - for example, a family of fishermen, builders etc).

The hereditary factor still has to be clarified and further epidemiological studies are required.

There are also environmental and individual risk factors that combine synergistically with the primary factors and have a certain degree of importance in prevention.

The risk factors can be split into two groups:

• Intrinsic factors

• Extrinsic factors

The intrinsic factors include hereditary factors, quantitative and qualitative alterations of the lac-rimal film and irritant chronic conjunctivitis.

Some deficiencies, such as the deficiency of Vitamin A, are responsible for an alteration of the lacrimal mucous layer and the corneal-conjunctival epithelial cell turnover and are considered to be intrinsic risk factors.

Race is an intrinsic risk factor whereas the geographical area is considered to be an extrinsic factor.

The extrinsic factors are largely exposure to UV light and chronic micro-trauma of the eye surface because of the patients profession.

The influence of exposure to micro-trauma in the work environment is unquestionable (allergens, wind, dust, smoke or other toxic stimuli), and farmers, sailors, carpenters, welders, builders are among the professional groups exposed to the greatest risk.[7, 9, 115, 116]

Microbial and viral infections would appear to be of secondary importance but in certain populations for example, trachoma competes in the secondary alteration of the lacrimal film and pre-disposes the conjunctiva to the damaging action of the environmental factors.

PRIMARY OR MAJOR RISK FACTORS

Intrinsic factors	Extrinsic factors
Hereditary (Not verified)	chronic exposure to UV radiation
Lacrimal alterations	micro-trauma to the eye
Vitamin A deficiency	microbial and viral infections
Race	
Solar keratosis	

Minor risk factors identified in the epidemiological studies include:[8,13,15,25,26]

- **Color of the eyes.** Green or hazel eyes would appear to be at a greater risk than brown eyes. Blue and gray eyes would appear to be at a minimal risk.

- **Skin pigmentation.** The people who tan easily when young run a lesser risk than the people who burn under the same conditions of sunlight exposure. Freckles on the skin of younger patients would appear to increase the risk of pterygium.

- **Solar keratosis.** There is a strong correlation between solar keratosis and pterygium.

- **Prevalence of pterygia** vary considerably in relation to the latitude.

- **Living environment.** Greater risk of pterygia has been observed if the patient lived his early years in a very sandy or dusty environment or living outdoors for more than 50% of the daylight hours, with exposure to solar radiation.

- **Sun filters.** Not wearing sun-glasses in very sunny climates increases the risk of pterygia.

4

ETIOLOGY

The biological and pathogenetic mechanisms that cause pterygia are not fully understood and the etiological theories proposed do not clarify the nature and origin of this lesion.

There is no clinical explanation for the erratic growth of the pterygium; spontaneous remission and sudden re-activation of growth are integral parts of the clinical evolution. It is unknown why some pterygia re-appear following removal, while others, of the same type, do not despite being subjected to the same treatment. It is not clear why there is uni-directional growth towards the center instead of growth that spreads over the entire surface and finally why growth stops when the head of the pterygium reaches the corneal apex. The pathogenetic theories have not provided a response to these questions and still cannot confirm whether the primary cause is a lesion of the limbal conjunctiva, damage to the peripheral cornea or damage to the limbus itself.

A summary of the etiological or pathogenetic theories follows:

- **Hereditary factors:** a pterygium, according to Sedan and Enroth is hereditary and is transmitted with a dominant gene of incomplete penetration. Hereditary factors are suspected because of an unusually high incidence in certain families down through a number of generations. According to the authors, the hereditary component refers to the predisposition of the conjunctiva to an abnormal reaction to atmospheric or environmental stimuli.[10,17,18]

- **Pinguecular:** this theory was suggested by

Fuchs and expanded by Guillermo Pico and others. These authors identified the primary lesion of the pterygium in the pinguecula;[2,6,9,10,51,113] micro-lesions at the limbus caused by environmental or lacrimal factors would provoke a defense reaction by the conjunctiva which would cause inflammatory cells to migrate to the conjunctiva with subsequent and spontaneous covering of the conjunctiva. The lesion, when it involves the cornea, produces edema which encourages the migration of limbal keratoblasts, the so-called "advancement front" of the lesion or "Fuchs' progressive area", visible in the superficial stroma of the cornea as cellular islets.

This theory was devised because of the histological similarity of the pterygium with pinguecula.

In support of the theory, Pico reports that a pinguecula is often observed in the fellow eye to pterygium. Contradicting this theory however, it should be reported that a pinguecula, despite being caused by environmental ultraviolet radiation, is common in regions, such as Japan, where a pterygium is rare.[4,115]

- **Inflammatory:** this theory has had numerous illustrious supporters in the past; Arlt, Scarpa, Hirschberg, Von Grafe, Kamel;[2,3,4,6,10,113] erosions and micro-ulcerations of the limbus provoked by environmental or professional stimuli could activate the conjunctiva with a sub-clinical inflammation to repair the lesion. In this theory, as in the pinguecular theory of Fuchs and Pico, the primary cause is the same.

- **Muscular:** according to this theory,[117] a pterygium originates from a degenerative reaction of the tendon of the medial rectus. It is a simplistic theory which provides no explanation for the type of degeneration or the appearance or progression of the pterygium.

- **Anomalies of the lacrimal film**: discontinuity of the lacrimal film with formation of small dellen and epithelial microulcerations. This would be the initial stimulation for the proliferation of the sub-conjunctival fibro-vascular tissue. Jose Barraquer (1958), without explaining the formation of the initial lesion at the limbus, emphasized the role played by the dry cornea in front of the head of the pterygium as a stimulus for its progression. A quantitative and qualitative alteration of the lacrimal film is therefore present in all pterygia.[19,20]

- **Tumoral:** this theory was proposed by d'Ombrain and Kamel[6,10,2] and suggests that the pterygium is a malignant tumor localized in the sub-conjunctival tissue. The hyperplastic fibrillary tissue would appear to be able to invade the cornea with active destruction of the epithelium, Bowman's and the stroma.

- **Neurotrophic:** Hervouet[117] proposed this theory. He suggested that the chronic irritation of the limbus creates neuritis of the corneal nerves in the nasal sector with consequent trophic ulceration. The repair of the limbal lesion through the bulbar conjunctiva, according to this theory, creates the primary lesion, and the subsequent scar retraction would create a localized discontinuity of the lacrimal film with ulceration of the limbus. This theory does not differ greatly from the suggestion of an inflammatory cause, and also includes the lacrimal theory suggested by Barraquer.[8,117,118]

- **Diet/nourishment:** according to Beard & Dimitry[10,119] a pterygium is caused by modifications of the epithelial trophism because of a deficiency of choline and Vitamin A. According to this theory, a pterygium is nothing more than a deficiency-linked epithelial dysplasia.

- **Angiogenetic tissue factors:** Wong, who devised this theory, suggested that repeated irritation of the limbus would produce an angiogenetic factor which would give rise to a pterygium. The angiogenetic factor, according to more recent studies,[22,119,120,121] could derive from corneal collagen protein denatured under the effects of ultraviolet light.

- **Virus:** the idea that a pterygium could be caused by a virus has been considered in the past[10] but a specific virus has never been isolated. Recently, in Africa, in geographical areas where pterygia are not endemic, the Papova virus was isolated in some patients affected by pterygia. However, this report has not been confirmed in other parts of the world.

- **Immunitary:** rather than being classed as a theory, this suggestion was made by Hilgers in the Sixties.[39]

  The author suggests a cell-mediated immunity unbalance in the conjunctiva. In the tissue excised from a pterygium, immunohistochemical techniques have highlighted a population of immunological cells with a prevalence of CD3 lymphocytes (with suppressor activity).[24,33,34] In the normal conjunctiva, the ratio between helper and suppressor cells normally lies at around 1:1.5. In pterygia, the mean ratio is 1:2.7.

  In addition to T lymphocytes, mastocytes, plasma cells and deposits of immunoglobulin with the characteristic granular pattern have been observed.

  The presence of IgE, IgG and immunological cells would seem to indicate that there are hypersensitivity immune reactions (types 1, 3 and 4) in a pterygium. It has not been clarified whether the immune reaction occurs in the phase of development or growth of the lesion, or whether it represents a response reaction to tissue damage. These observations deserve further investigation to clarify whether immune mechanisms are involved in the definition of the clinical behavior of a pterygium or whether it is an immune reaction associated to secondary degenerative phenomena.

- **Environmental ultraviolet lighting:** this is currently the most credible theory. It hypothesizes the appearance of a pterygium because of the cumulative effect of UV absorbed by the eye surface. The UV light causes histological alterations in the epithelial cells and in the sub-mucosal conjunctival tissue[11,12,18] and would appear to be responsible for other chronic pathologies of the conjunctiva and the cornea.[13,14,15,22,25,26] UV radiation between 290 and 320 nm is absorbed selectively by the epithelial and sub-epithelial layers of the eye surface. The photo-toxic effect of UV light is greater for UVA and the damage caused by these rays can be incremented by the presence of endogenic and exogenic psoralenic substances which by means of their photo-sensitizing activity, accentuate the UV damage.[21] The single high doses of UV cause acute actinic keratoconjunctivitis with the well-known clinical picture of corneal and conjunctival epithelium sloughing which is very painful. On the other hand, the chronic daily doses of UV light can permanently damage the eye surface producing degeneration of Bowman's membrane and the superficial stromal lamellae and may even provoke a fine peripheral network of neo-vascularization in the stroma.[27] Because of its particular spherical shape and its radius of curvature, the cornea reacts in an unusual manner to the light incident on its surface. Part of the incident light is focused on the retina by the dioptric structures, and part is scattered in the stroma. It has been demonstrated that the scattering of light originating from the corneal surface and the stroma is concentrated largely at the limbus, up to 20 times more than in the remainder of the cornea. The light incident on the temporal side of the cornea is concentrated at the nasal side, while the light incident on the nasal sector concentrates to a lesser degree at the temporal limbus because of interference by the nose. This phenomenon, demonstrated with a mathematical model, is more evident in corneas with greater curvature where the concentration of light at the limbus is greater than in flatter corneas.[28,29,30] This phenomenon may also explain the greater frequency of a pterygium at the nasal limbus.

- **Limbal theory:** until recent years, the limbus was simply considered to be a transition zone between the cornea, the sclera and the conjunctiva, that is, an anatomical region without a specific function. In recent years, numerous studies have proved that the limbus actually possesses important activities of regulation and proliferation of the corneal epithelium and can act as a barrier against stimuli and pathologies originating in the conjunctiva. There are no sure elements that support the fact that the limbus is the starting point of metabolic stimuli that can activate a mechanism of proliferation such as a pterygium, but there is indirect proof that points to limbal damage as the primary cause of a pterygium.

The indirect proof is the clinical observation that in the surgical treatment of pterygium, the treatment of the conjunctival component often causes re-appearance of a pterygium while the limbal treatment, which restores a certain degree of barrier function, will provide better therapeutic results. Immuno-histochemistry, using monoclonal antibodies specific for the cytokeratine of the epithelial cells of the conjunctiva and the cornea, would appear to suggest that the pterygium originates from the stem cells of the limbus;[32] these cells are normally fixed but possibly under the effect of etiological environmental factors (UV) or other local influences, and through the effect of tissue mediators, they give rise to daughter cells that can migrate below the basal membrane of the conjunctival and corneal epithelium (migrant keratoblasts).

During their advancement towards the cornea, these cells can damage and destroy Bowman's membrane and can infiltrate the superficial stromal lamellae.

During their migration, the keratoblasts do not possess any fibroblastic activity but acquire it at the end of the migration.

5

HISTOLOGY

There are numerous histological alterations in a pterygium and they involve both the conjunctiva and the cornea, but none is specific to a pterygium.

Histological studies completed to evaluate the existence of cell or tissue markers that can differentiate stationary from recurrent pterygium[41] have not highlighted any differentiating characteristics.

CONJUNCTIVA

This epithelium presents the histological alterations more precociously. New cylindrical cell layers are observed intercalated with muciferous calciform cells which insinuate in the numerous folds and troughs in a pterygium to create cystic gland-like structures.

At the head of pterygium, there is a sharp transition between conjunctival and corneal epithelium and the epithelial cells of the cornea assume a "lumpy" appearance.

Impression cytology[35] has shown that the epithelium covering the pterygium presents a certain degree of atrophy and phenomena of metaplasia, compared to the healthy conjunctiva around it.

The conjunctival substance would appear to become involved at a later stage with phenomena of degeneration and fragmentation of the elastic fibers and hyaline degeneration of the peri-limbal connective tissue.[25,26,27]

In a pterygium, in comparison to the healthy conjunctiva, the glycosaminoglycans (GAG) of the interstitial substance show a significant increase in hydroxyproline[36] and a reduction in the enzymes necessary for the production of the interstitial substance.[37]

In both the normal conjunctiva and in pterygia, collagen type I, II and III are present.

However, collagen type II is not present in the cornea and the fact that it is found in pterygium would suggest conjunctival genesis of this pathology, at least where the superficial component is concerned.

CORNEA

The earliest alterations in the cornea are seen in Bowman's membrane where small vesicles are observed at the entrance point of the nerves to the sub-epithelial plexus.

In an advanced pterygium, where there is greater corneal involvement, Bowman's membrane is destroyed for the entire extension of the pterygium with the exception of 1-2 mm beyond the apex.

There are numerous fissures in the superficial lamellae of the corneal stroma with degeneration of the elastic fibers and hyaline degeneration of the collagen fibers. It is not unusual to find "glove finger" histological images in the stroma, as described by Hervouet in 1954; these are islets of conjunctival epithelium that are embedded in depth forming small cysts.

These epithelial islets can be observed at the slit lamp and are referred to as Fuch's patches.

Histological Differences in the Various Evolutionary Phases of Pterygia

There are histological differences between the various phases of development of pterygium. In a stationary pterygium, the sub-epithelial fibrous component stops precisely at the apex of the pterygium, perpendicularly or at the slightly oblique edges, and the fibrils appear irregular or disintegrated. The histological aspect of an advanced pterygium is characterized by the presence of a large amount of fibrous tissue which replaces Bowman's membrane, and in the more superficial layers of the stroma, the basal membrane of the epithelium rests directly on the fibrous layer of the pterygium.

Cytology in a Pterygium

The cellular component in a pterygium consists of fibroblasts and immunity cells: T lymphocytes (CD3), monocytes, plasma cells, macrophages and mastocytes.[40]

The primary culture of fibroblasts from the pterygium highlighted some atypical behavior compared to the fibroblasts in healthy conjunctiva.

In a pterygium, the fibroblast culture showed a reduced dependency on growth factors and a more rapid saturation of the culture.[38]

This indicates active proliferation of the lesion.

6
CLINICAL ANATOMY

The bulbar conjunctiva of the medial canthus is the preferred site for pterygium (91%). In 25% of patients both eyes are affected but it is rare for two lesions to form in the same eye *(Figures 6-1, 6-2)*. A temporal position is possible.

Certain morphological and anatomical features of pterygium can be identified by slit lamp examination which allow the pathology to be differentiated and classed in its various clinical forms. Over the years and as the pathology progresses, a pterygium undergoes a number of morphological changes that allow the eye surgeon to evaluate whether the situation is stationary or whether there has been further growth.

Awareness of these clinical aspects is extremely important in the management of a pterygium because it allows the clinical forms to be classed and the prognosis, within certain limits, in terms of evolution and treatment which may provide the best therapeutic outcome.

If we start from the cornea and move towards the conjunctiva, we can identify:

- **The hood:** this precedes the head of a pterygium on the cornea. It appears as a half-moon shaped grayish avascular patch on the corneal epithelium around the apex *(Figures 6-3, 6-4)*. At the hood, when a pterygium is active, there are numerous micro-ulcerations of the epithelium which can be stained with fluorescein. The underlying stroma appears cloudy. When a pterygium is stationary, the epithelium is not stained with fluorescein and the stroma appears clear.

- **Fuchs' patches:** these appear as small irregular areas of grayish opacity in front of the hood and under the corneal epithelium. In the active phase, because of the epithelial micro-ulcerations of the hood and the infiltration of the underlying stroma, Fuchs' patches cannot be clearly observed. On the other hand, in the stationary forms these opaque areas are clearly defined and covered by intact epithelium *(Figures 6-7, 6-8, 6-9)*.

- **Stocker's line:** this is a fine yellow-green half-moon-shaped line in front of the head. It is formed by the accumulation of hemosiderine at Bowman's membrane. Stocker's line is a morphological marker of a chronic lesion and indicates that in recent years a pterygium has not progressed. Stocker's line is evident in many stationary pterygia; however, in a rapidly evolving pterygium it does not have time to form *(Figure 6-10)*.

- **Apex or head:** this is the portion of the pterygium that invades the cornea. Generally speaking it is white, raised and attached firmly to the underlying cornea *(Figure 6-11)*. In the stationary forms, it is whitish, raised very slightly and with almost negligible vascularization *(Figure 6-10)*. In an advanced pterygium, the apex protrudes from the eye surface and is vascularized with indented edges and small capillaries anastomized with the limbal plexus *(Figure 6-12)*.

- **The collarette or collar:** this is observed in all pterygia and is the limbal portion of the lesion. Of varying extension, it is continuous with the body.

- **The body:** this is a fold or a strip of highly vascularized tissue. It is normally trapezoidal in shape and it extends medially as far as the semi-lunar fold. The vessels of the body form a straight line as though they have been stretched. There is a natural cleavage plane with the underlying episcleral tissue. The color and appearance of the body of the pterygium changes in the various clinical phases. In the stationary forms it is only slightly raised and appears as a pink strip of fine, straight capillaries *(Figures 6-10, 6-11, 6-14)* while in the active phase it is bright red or livid due to the conjunctival vascularization and the underlying fibro-vascular tissue. There are a number of capillaries that are dilated and anastomosed to each other.

- **The edges:** these are created from conjunctival folds that define the boundary between the body of a pterygium and the surrounding conjunctiva. These may be raised slightly in an advanced pterygium, and fine in the initial or stationary forms.

The two tables that follow summarize the morphological variations of pterygia in the various clinical situations.

STATIONARY PTERIGIUM	
Hood	Non-vascular half-moon grayish opacity of the epithelium that cannot be stained with fluorescein.
Fuchs spots	Clearly visible as small irregular grayish zones in front of the head in the sub-epithelium, in the superficial stroma.
Stocker Line	Visible as a yellow/brownish half-moon shaped line in front of the head; it indicates how chronic the pathology is.
Apex or head	Whitish, minimally raised and poorly vascularized.
Body	Minimally raised, pearly white or pinkish in color. Poor vascularization with visible episcleral vessels.

ACTIVE OR EVOLVING PTERYGIUM	
Hood	There are epithelial micro-ulcerations that can be stained with fluorescein. The underlying stroma is usually cloudy.
Fuchs spots	These are not clearly visible because of the epithelial micro-ulcerations and because of the cloudiness of the hood.
Stocker line	A rapidly growing pterygium will not allow the Stocker line to form.
Apex or head	This is raised and highly vascularized; small capillaries are visible that have anastomized with the limbal plexus.
Body	The color is bright red or livid, it is thick and raised, and has a fleshy appearance because of the numerous dilated and congested capillaries

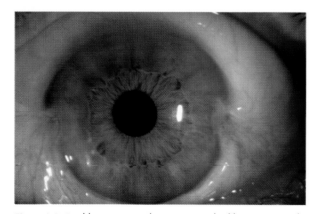

Figure 6-1. *Double pterygium. The patient's medical history reports the almost simultaneous appearance of a pterygium in both eyes with associated inflammation. The patient has a number of risk factors and a family history of pterygia.*

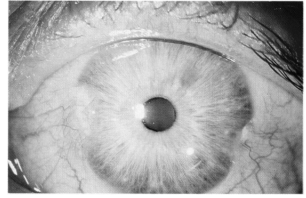

Figure 6-2. *Double pterygium. The patient is a 54-year-old brick-layer with a family history of pterygia (his father and two younger brothers were affected). A nasal pterygium is normally more advanced than the temporal.*

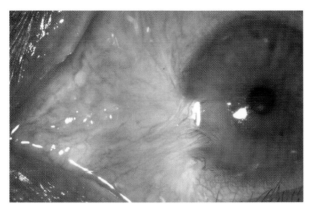

Figure 6-3. *Stationary pterygium. The hood of the pterygium is visible as a grayish cloudy non-vascular zone of the corneal epithelium surrounding the head of the pterygium. In a progressive pterygium, there are epithelial micro-ulcerations that are absent in the stationary forms. The epithelium does not stain and the stroma is transparent.*

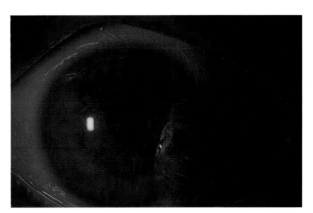

Figure 6-6. *Pterygium in the active phase. Again the patient of figure 6-5 following staining with fluorescein. The staining highlights the epithelial damage and the corneal micro-ulcerations in front of the head of the pterygium.*

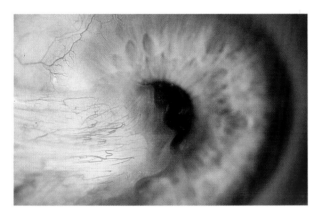

Figure 6-4. *Stationary pterygium. The hood is clearly visible as a festooned gray band in front of the head of the pterygium. In the zones of relative opacity, there are no signs of epithelial damage and some Fuchs patches are clearly visible.*

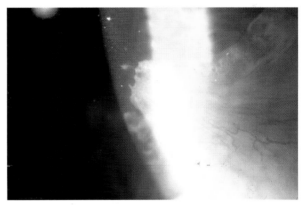

Figure 6-7. *Stationary pterygium. The Fuchs patches are visible as small grayish areas distributed unevenly in front of the head of the pterygium and under the corneal epithelium of the superficial stroma. In the stationary forms, the outline is very clear whereas during the phases of activation, the Fuchs patches are not very obvious because of the cloudiness of the stroma and the epithelial damage.*

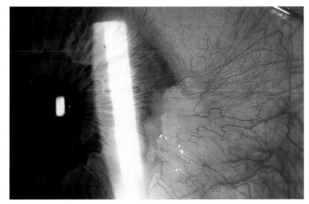

Figure 6-5. *Pterygium in the active phase. The hood of the pterygium is visible as an irregular grayish line in front of the head with clouding of the underlying corneal stroma and damage of the surrounding epithelium.*

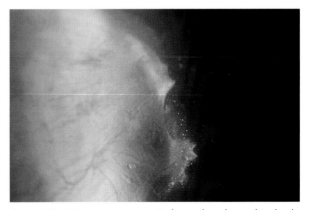

Figure 6-8. *Stationary pterygium. Fuchs patches observed under the highest magnification of the slit lamp. The overlying corneal epithelium is intact and permits good vision.*

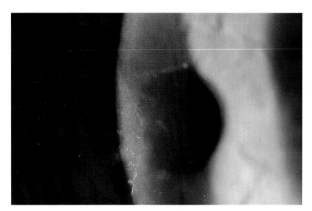

Figure 6-9. *Activation of pterygium. Following many stationary years, the pterygium has re-activated. The collarette and the superficial stroma become cloudy. The infiltration and the stromal cloudiness reduce visibility of the Fuchs patches, the edges of which are not as clearly visible as before.*

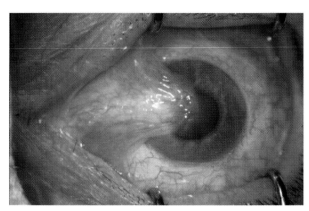

Figure 6-12. *Active pterygium. The color of the body of the pterygium is bright red, almost livid, it is thickened and has a meaty appearance because of the congestion of the dilated blood vessels. There are micro-ulcerations of the epithelium in the hood, and the underlying and surrounding stroma is cloudy.*

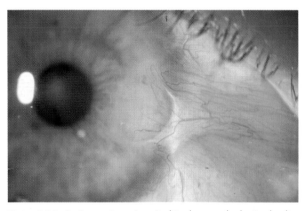

Figure 6-10. *Stationary Pterygium. In this photograph, the Stocker line is just visible as a fine, half-moon-shaped yellow-green line in front of the head of the pterygium. The Stocker line is formed by an accumulation of hemosiderine at Bowman's layer and is a morphological marker of how chronic the lesion has become. The body consists of a fine band of fine, straight capillaries.*

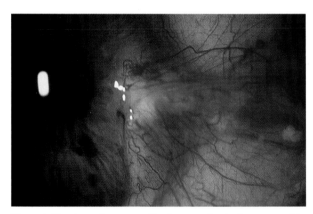

Figure 6-13. *Active Pterygium. The hypertrophic body is crossed by numerous injected capillaries that are anastomosed to each other. There is poor proliferation of the sub-conjunctival tissue and the episclera vessels can be observed.*

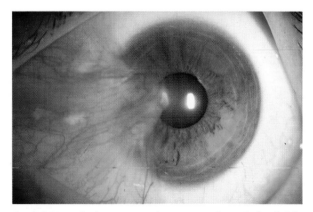

Figure 6-11. *Evolved pterygium in the stationary phase. The head of the pterygium appears as a whitish, poorly vascularized band which invades the pupillary space and is strongly adherent to the underlying cornea. There are no clinical signs of activation. In the body, the sub-conjunctival fibrosis is obvious and extends as far as the semilunar fold.*

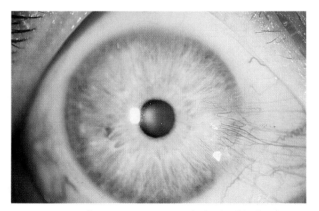

Figure 6-14. *Small stationary pterygium. The body of the lesion is not highly vascularized and the edges blend progressively with the surrounding healthy conjunctiva. There is very little sub-conjunctival fibro-vascular tissue and the episcleral vessels can be observed.*

7

CLINICAL PICTURE
AND CLASSIFICATION

The morphological features of pterygia and the involvement of the cornea lead to the classification of some clinical forms. There are three main types. The groups of classification can be split on the basis of the evolution and the severity of the clinical picture - from the initial forms to the more advanced stages.

The clinical features considered in this classification are: size, vascularization, the extension on the corneal surface, the involvement of the optical zone and the complications.

SMALL PRIMARY PTERYGIUM (Type 1)

This includes the initial stages of a primary pteygium that are poorly evolved. These lesions are restricted to the limbus or only marginally invade the cornea. In these forms, the symptoms and the complications are almost absent as these are stationary forms with very slow clinical evolution.

The morphology at the slit lamp highlights three different types of pterygia

- *Fibrous.* The pterygium appears as a small whitish or yellowish ring that is parallel to the limbus with conjunctival blood vessels that converge towards it. The body is not clearly seen as it is lost in the surrounding healthy conjunctiva *(Figures 7-1, 7-2).*

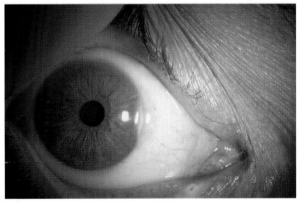

Figure 7-1. *Pterygium Type I with fibrous appearance. This small stationary pterygium has a very slightly raised head at the limbus, and resembles a small whitish fibrous ring that is poorly vascularized. The body is barely visible, and blends progressively with the surrounding healthy conjunctiva.*

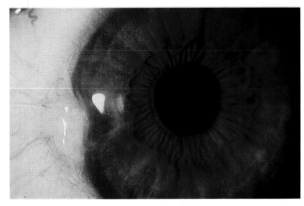

Figure 7-2. *Primary pterygium Type I with fibrous appearance. Compared to the previous picture, we can observe major involvement of the cornea and a certain degree of irregularity of the surrounding corneal epithelium caused by poor distribution of the lacrimal film.*

- *Pinguecular.* A pterygium has an appearance similar to a pinguecula. It is raised with respect to the limbus and the head does not invade the cornea which appears to be infiltrated by the stroma in a small area of 2-3 mm. The body consists of a slight horizontal vascularization at the medial canthus which is often difficult to distinguish from the surrounding healthy conjunctiva (*Figure 7-3*).

- *Classical.* This is the classical form of a pterygium where the various portions are clearly defined: head or apex, collarette and edges, body. The apex invades the cornea for about 1-2 mm (*Figure 7-4*). This third type is observed in just slightly more than one third of all cases of Type I pterygia.

ADVANCED PRIMARY OR RECURRENT PTERYGIUM WITH NO OPTICAL ZONE INVOLVEMENT *(Type II)*

This is the most common type and includes both primary and recurrent forms. In this pterygium it is possible to distinguish all the anatomical structures clearly. The head is raised and invades the cornea as far as the optic zone; the surrounding infiltrated area is visible to the naked eye. The body is crossed by dilated capillaries that form a vascularized band which fans out at the internal canthus. Irritation is constant in these patients and any reduction in vision is caused by induced astigmatism or by light diffraction phenomena (*Figures 7-5, 7-6, 7-7, 7-8, 7-9, 7-10*).

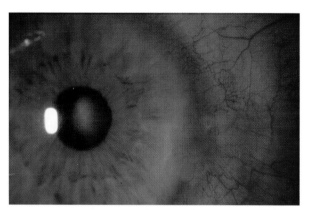

Figure 7-3. *Pterygium Type I with pinguecular appearance. The lesion is raised compared to the limbus and the head does not invade the cornea which appears to be invaded for about 2 mm. The body is vascularized and shows a certain degree of capillary congestion.*

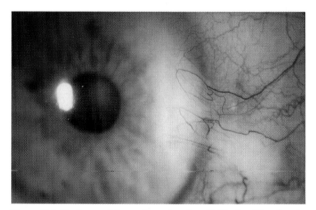

Figure 7-5. *Stationary Primary Pterygium Type II. The head involves the cornea and is surrounded by an area of stromal infiltration. Some major and minor vessels can be seen in the barely raised body.*

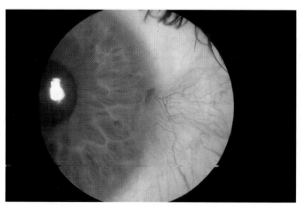

Figure 7-4. *Pterygium Type I with classical appearance. The various parts are clearly visible: head, collarette, edges and body. The head involves the cornea for about 1-2 mm. The minor hemorrhage indicates the activity of the pterygium.*

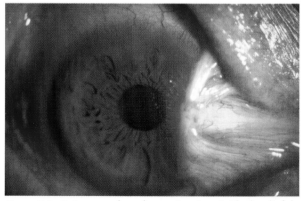

Figure 7-6. *Stationary, relapsed pterygium Type II. The head of the lesion shows no clinical signs of activity even though the stromal infiltration and the irregularity produce irregular astigmatism with a reduction in vision. The body of the pterygium is not highly vascularized but consists of abundant sub-conjunctival fibrous tissue which causes anatomical damage to the structures of the medial canthus and in the conjunctival fornices with symblepharon formation.*

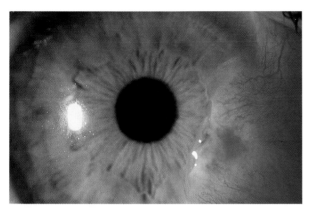

Figure 7-7. *Progressive primary pterygium Type II. At the slit lamp, the signs of activation are clear; the head is raised and highly vascularized with injected, congested capillaries and minor hemorrhage. The head is surrounded by an area of cloudy stroma and by epithelial micro-ulcerations. The body resembles a large reddish band of injected capillaries.*

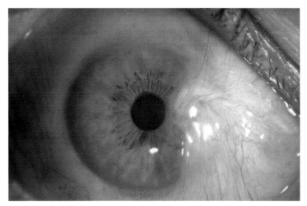

Figure 7-10. *Stationary recurrent pterygium Type II. The head of the pterygium has not invaded the optical zone but the vision is reduced because of the severe irregular astigmatism. In the body, sub-conjunctival fibrosis predominates which produces diplopia because of infiltration of the sheath of the medial rectus tendon which reduces abduction of the globe.*

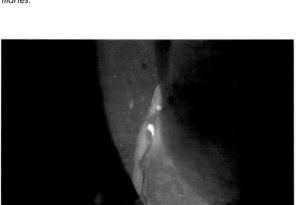

Figure 7-8. *The same case shown in Figure 7-7, this time stained with fluorescein. Observe the epithelial damage caused by micro-ulcerations in front of the head of the pterygium.*

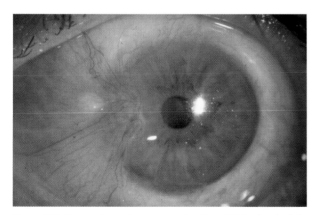

Figure 7-9. *Progressive primary pterygium Type II. The head of the pterygium appears to be raised and highly vascularized; around the head, there is infiltration of the stroma with epithelial micro-ulcerations. The body is not particularly hypertrophic but is considerably extensive.*

ADVANCED PRIMARY OR RECURRENT PTERYGIUM WITH OPTICAL ZONE INVOLVEMENT *(Type III)*

This is the most advanced form of pterygium. The invasion of the optical zone is the distinguishing feature in this group of pterygia. The growth of this pterygium is such that the apex invades the pupillary field and the infiltration of the stroma involves at least 30% of the corneal thickness.

The reduction in vision is always evident and caused by astigmatism and involvement of the optical zone.

The morphological features of Type III pterygia are:

- the obvious collarette which can extend for 8-10 mm in the limbus,

- a considerably developed body with a prevalence of a very strong sub-conjunctival fibrous component. In certain cases this may adhere to the capsule which surrounds the tendon of the medial rectus muscle and limit the abduction of the globe; alternately, in the conjunctival fornices, it may create symblepharon - like scarring or ectropion of the inferior lacrimal punctum.

Type III pterygia also includes the rapidly evolving forms and the violent post-operative recurrences that are labeled with the term "malignant pterygium" *(Figures 7-11, 7-12, 7-13, 7-14, 7-15, 7-16).*

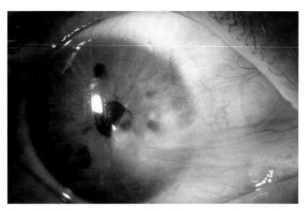

Figure 7-11. *Stationary recurrent Type III pterygium. The optical zone is invaded by a strip of opacity that creates considerable irregularity of the optical zone and severe astigmatism. The apex of the pterygium stops before and is firmly adherent to the cornea. The body appears to be poorly vascularized and the sub-conjunctival fibrous component is poor, allowing glimpses of some episcleral vessels.*

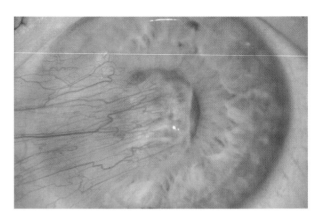

Figure 7-14. *Primary pterygium Type III. The head of the pterygium has completely invaded the pupillary space reducing vision to hand-movement. In the body, the central vessels of the pterygium are clearly visible; however, the amount of fibrosis is not particularly abundant.*

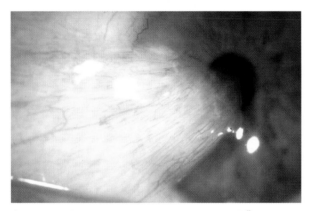

Figure 7-12. *Stationary primary pterygium Type III. Following many years of slow, progressive growth reported by the patient, the lesion has stopped progressing. In the optical zone, the hood is clearly visible and appears as an irregular area of opacity of the stromal surface. An accumulation of hemosiderin indicates that the progression of the pterygium has stopped and that the lesion is clinically stable.*

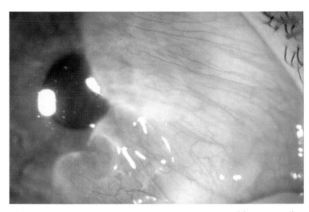

Figure 7-15. *Recurrent pterygium Type III. A 46-year-old patient with a family history of pterygia and numerous professional risk factors. There is considerable expansion of the head of the pterygium on the cornea and the extension of the collarette to the limbus reaches 13 mm. There is abundant and tenacious sub-conjunctival fibrosis, with diplopia in lateral gaze due to the infiltration of the medial rectus muscle.*

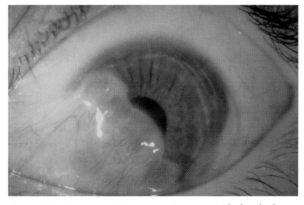

Figure 7-13. *Stationary primary pterygium Type III. The head is hypertrophic and protrudes considerably from the corneal plane. The optical zone is irreparably invaded and vision has dropped to 2/10 with a pin-hole. The sub-conjunctival fibrous component of the body is considerable because of symblepharon of the superior fornix.*

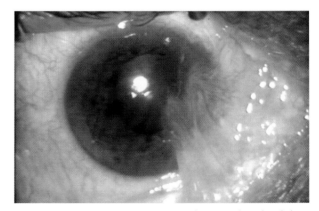

Figure 7-16. *Recurrent pterygium Type III. The patient has already been subjected to six operations for the simple removal of a pterygium and the recurrences have always been constant and rapid. In this case, the recurrence appeared with unusual violence just a few days after the last operation. This type of clinical progression is considered malignant.*

Table summarizing the clinical classification of pterygium

TYPE I

Initial forms of pterygia. Very mild or no symptoms.

Fibrous: small whitish or yellowish circles parallel to the limbus.
Conjunctival blood vessels converging towards the circles.
The body is not clearly distinguished.

Pinguecular: appearance is similar to pinguecula, protruding.
The head can just about be identified and does not invade the cornea; there is 2-3 mm of stromal infiltration.

Classical: all the portions can be clearly identified. The apex invades 1-2 mm of the cornea.

TYPE II - PRIMARY OR RECURRENT

Irritation and initial reduction in vision due to irregular astigmatism. The cornea is invaded for 2-4 mm and reaches the optical zone. The body is thickened with dilated, congested capillaries. The corneal infiltration can be seen with the naked eye.

TYPE III - VERY ADVANCED OR "MALIGNANT" RECURRENT PTERYGIUM

Obvious symptoms with serious reduction in vision. There may be oculo-motory disturbances and a watery eye syndrome. The head invades the cornea for more than 4 mm and reaches the optical zone. There is always a reduction in vision, the collarette is extended (up to 8-10 mm) and the body extends for the entire medial canthus. There is abundant sub-conjunctival fibrosis which extends as far as the fornices.

8

CLINICAL EVOLUTION

As the origin and the evolution of pterygia are still not clear, the eye surgeon will be faced with a number of questions:

1. What are the initial signs of pterygia?
2. Can the evolution be predicted on the basis of the onset?
3. Can a pterygium develop from pinguecula?
4. When should the surgeon wait and for how long, and when should he intervene?

The origin and nature of the primary pterygium lesion is still not fully understood. According to some authors,[116] the transition from the primary lesion to the full-blown form occurs with the appearance of small grayish opaque areas in the corneal stroma close to the nasal limbus (Fuchs area), but the primary lesion has not been described with details of the clinical and morphological features.

According to Cornand,[55,111] the development of pterygium occurs in two successive phases:

1 - Conjunctival or pre-pterygium phase
2 - Corneal or true pterygium phase

The conjunctival stage appears in the second decade of life and manifests itself as irritation, burning, hyperemia and foreign body sensation. The disturbances are reported as discontinuous and worsen on exposure to sunlight, dust and wind.

The objective examination highlights conjunctival hyperemia localized in the medial canthus and moderate conjunctival and sub-conjunctival edema. The capillaries of the nasal conjunctiva are dilated and twisted.

Staining with fluorescein or preferably with 1% Bengal rose demonstrates signs of wide-spread sloughing of the conjunctival epithelium.

The possible clinical evolution of these lesions is as follows:

a) formation of a raised pinguecula at the nasal limbus;
b) formation, close to the limbus, of a small raised fibrous ring that is poorly vascularized. This is caused by the repair and scarring of the conjunctiva at the nasal limbus. The ring creates a circumscribed discontinuity of the lacrimal film which causes corneal micro-ulcerations and accentuates the irritation.[8] The repair of these micro-ulcerations stimulates the invasion of new blood vessels and permits the progression of the conjunctiva towards the cornea with the formation of pterygium.

The possibility of predicting the clinical evolution of pterygia on the basis of the onset is another question which has not been answered to date. Pterygia normally grows very slowly but the growth rate is unpredictable. Having said this, cases have been reported of forms that stopped growing completely following years of progression.[8] Generally speaking, following a growth or active phase, the appearance of a pterygium changes; the lesion becomes pale, initially at the head and followed by the body with a considerable reduction in thickness; the capillaries are less injected, the central vessels disappear.

In the forms that re-appear following surgery, progression may be rapid and sometimes violent, and occurs the so-called malignant forms. This may greatly compromise the optical zone.[117,122]

It is still not clear whether a pinguecula is a stage that precedes the development of a pterygium.

Fuchs, Pico and many other authors have identified pinguecula as the conjunctival lesion that gives rise to a pterygium.[2,6,9,10,51,113] This theory is based on the fact that, histologically, the two lesions are very similar.

At the time this writing, the two lesions are considered to be separate pathologies but with a common etiology: environmental ultraviolet radiation; pinguecula, like pterygium, affects people who are subjected to chronic exposure to sunlight and environmental micro-trauma.

A pinguecula is also common in areas where a pterygium is a rare occurrence, Japan for example[4,115] and it can affect the temporal sector of the limbus; it does not re-appear if removed for aesthetic reasons.

In some rare cases, the evolution of a pterygium does not follow the normal pattern and the unusual clinical picture produced may be serious. The surgeon should be aware of this possibility and be in a position to recognize the condition. Spontaneous sub-conjunctival hemorrhages are a rare occurrence, and almost always present in the active phases. An equally rare occurrence is the cystic transformation from epithelial folds that remain inside the fibro-vascular tissue of the pterygium. These give rise to pseudo-cystic formations that may become pigmented in time through oxidation *(Figure 8-1)*.

The epithelial epidermoid metaplasia is a pre-cancerous evolution where the surface epithelium takes on a pseudo-epithelial appearance.

The cancerous degeneration is the most serious form of evolution. It is a very rare occurrence in the Western civilizations but is observed in 1%-1.5% of pterygia in tropical or sub-tropical zones where pterygia are endemic.[4]

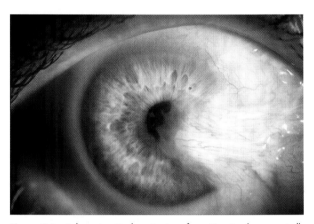

Figure 8-1. *Sub-conjunctival cystic transformation in the repeatedly recurrent pterygium. At the medial canthus, we can observe the yellowish cystic formation provoked by the oxidation of sub-conjunctival epithelial pseudo-cysts.*

9

SYMPTOMS

The severity of the symptoms of a pterygium are directly proportional to the clinical picture. In Pterygium Type I, symptoms are almost absent or of modest entity. However, in the more advanced forms, irritation is always reported and vision is always compromised.

The reduction of vision is a disturbance, varying with pterygium Type II and Type III; in these cases the head of the pterygium causes irregular astigmatism or invades the optical zone.

The irritation is non-specific: photophobia, a burning sensation on exposure to cold and heat, a foreign body sensation with sporadic or continual weeping.

The symptoms are accentuated during the "inflammatory" phases of pterygium and are associated with pain provoked by the corneal micro-ulcerations around the head of the pterygium.

A reduction in vision is observed when the growth of the pterygium on the cornea exceeds 3-4 mm; however, disturbances of vision are also reported in less evolved situations.

` Prior to a reduction in vision, the patient complains of generic disturbances of glare described as difficulty with night-driving or as "radiated" light effects. This disturbance is frequent, even with small dimension pterygia, and caused by a reduction in contrast sensitivity.

There is no linear correlation between the degree of glare and the corneal extension of the pterygium[42,43] and the tests to measure the contrast threshold under luminous stress have proved positive in all patients affected by the pathology, though the degree may differ:[44] the reduction mainly in-

volves the moderate/low spatial frequencies.

In the normal cornea, the lacrimal film is uniform and the lamellae and the fibers of the stroma are regular. This provides optimal physical condition for clear image reproduction with the simultaneous presence of these factors preventing the light incident on the cornea from being diffracted.

In a pterygium, due to the peripheral corneal opacities and alterations of the lacrimal film, there is greater diffraction of the incident light and contrast sensitivity is reduced.

Diffraction and alterations of vision appear and can be observed when the pupil diameter reaches and exceeds 6 mm; diameters of between 2-4 mm will not be affected.

Reduction of vision in pterygia is provoked essentially by two factors: induced astigmatism and invasion of the optical zone.

Astigmatism in pterygia is caused by a number of factors which can act independently or in association.[47,48,49]

The growth of the head of a pterygium on the cornea always creates a deformation in the corneal curvature.

A mathematical model examined the static and dynamic forces produced on the corneal curvature[45] and calculated that a pterygium produces a constant vector force when the adhesion at the insertion points is uniform. It also calculated that the deformation equals that produced by a weight of 5 grams for every mm of cornea involved.

In the cases of a pterygium where fibrous tissue creates strong adhesions with the structures of the medial canthus, in addition to the static deformation, there is the additional traction effect at the extreme points of vision.

In these cases, a pterygium produces a dynamic vector force which varies in intensity in relation to globe movements.

The static deformation acts in a single direction and the variations in curvature of the cornea do not affect the entire meridian but only the semi-meridian producing irregular and asymmetric astigmatism.

Dynamic deformation is caused by the movement of the globe, abduction in particular; and in very advanced pterygia, this deformation can be observed at the slit lamp as fine striae of the Descemet's space membrane, visible when the patient is asked to look in a direction opposite to position of the pterygium, or from comparative maps with Computerized Corneal Topography (CCT) with the examination performed in the primary and eccentric positions.

CCT is proving to be an extremely useful examination in the semeiotics of a pterygium because it permits the changes in corneal curvature induced by the pterygium to be evaluated, and provides useful information on the types of astigmatism, the extension of the deformation, and by using differential maps, the changes induced by surgery.[48]

In highly advanced pterygia, and particularly in a recurrence, there may be a symblepharon circumscribing the medial canthus and restrictions of globe abduction with diplopia in lateral gaze. This is rare in primary pterygia, but more frequent in recurrences consequent to repeated excision surgery.

These complications are caused by the proliferation of sub-conjunctival fibrovascular tissue that create strong adhesions with the connective tissue of the fornices and with the tendon capsular expansions of the medial rectus muscle (*Figures 9-1, 9-2*).

In the more serious cases, there may also be moderate enophthalmos at the extremes of gaze. It should also be remembered that, with the same mechanism, in some serious forms of pterygia, there may be an ectropion or entropion of the lacrimal puncta with persistent weeping.

Map 1: OD: Topographical picture of primary pterygium Type I, with 1.5 mm corneal involvement.
There is moderate irregularity in the optical zone and in the nasal sector of the cornea, linked to an alteration of the lacrimal film.

Map 2: OD: Primary pterygium Type II non-evolutive. The head invades 2.5 mm of the cornea. There is regular astigmatism.
Vod = 20/20 + 0.25 sph + 1.25 cyl at 75°
Vos = 20/22 + 0.25 sph + 1.25 cyl at 140°

Map 3: OS: Primary pterygium Type II evolutive
The head invades about 3 mm of the cornea, but at the collarette, there are signs of epithelial sloughing and a discontinuity of the lacrimal film.

The induced astigmatism is irregular.
Vod = 20/22 without correction
Vos = 20/22-25 + 0.25 sph + 2.50 cyl 80°

Map 4: OS: Keratoscopic picture of a primary pterygium Type III. The optical zone is marginally invaded by the head of the pterygium. The optical zone is considerably altered because of the corneal infiltration and the irregularity of the lacrimal film.
Vos = 20/66-100 -1.50 sph + 2.75 cyl at 105°

Map 5: OS: The same patient as Map 4, six months after peripheral lamellar keratoplasty.
The optical zone is now regular. Regular astigmatism of 1.81 D persists.
Postop. VOS = 20/25 - 1.25 cyl at 110°

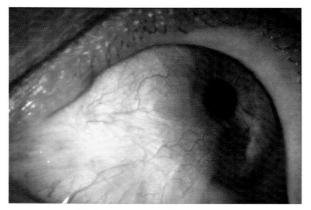

Figure 9-1. *Symblepharon in repeatedly recurrent Type II pterygium. In this patient, numerous operations of simple excision have provoked the proliferation of highly tenacious sub-conjunctival fibrous tissue that has invaded the conjunctival fornix at the medial canthus provoking a scar symblepharon and a reduction in abduction with diplopia in lateral gaze.*

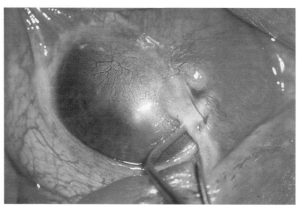

Figure 9-2. *Repeatedly recurrent pterygium Type III. This pterygium has been operated on numerous occasions with techniques of simple excision and has developed fibrous proliferation that has extensively invaded the cornea and all the anatomical structures of the medial canthus. In addition to diplopia, the eye has developed enophthalmus.*

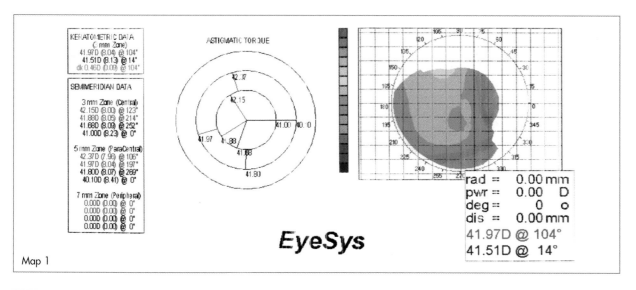

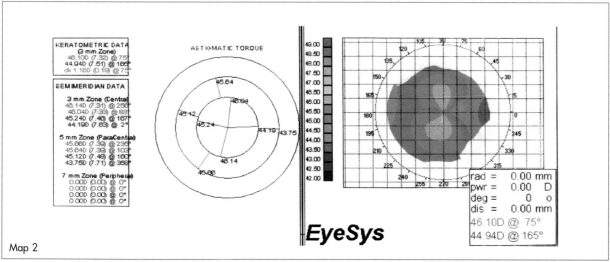

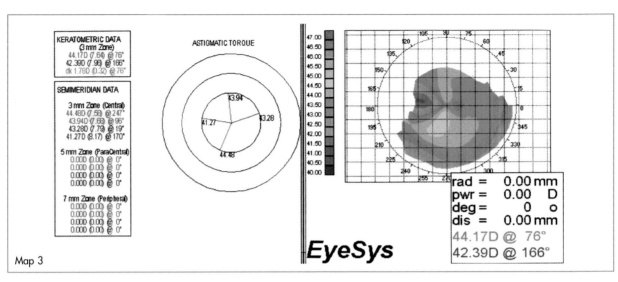

Map 3

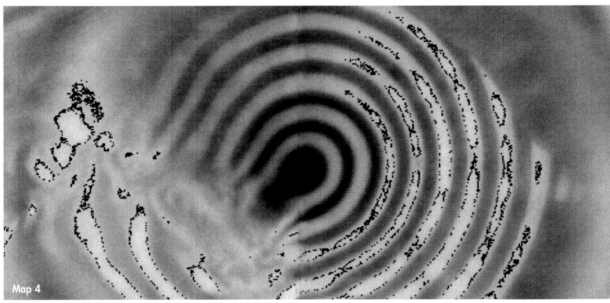

Map 4

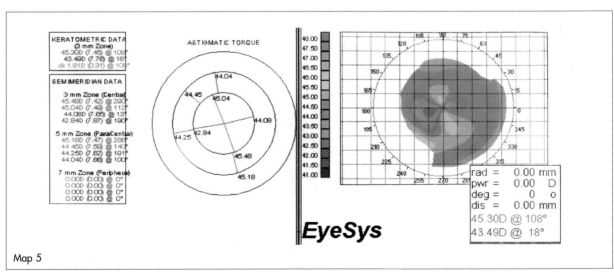

Map 5

10

DIFFERENTIAL DIAGNOSIS

Pterygia have a typical appearance at the slit lamp and diagnosis is rarely difficult.

However, some pathologies of the peripheral cornea and the limbus have a morphological appearance similar to pterygia. As a result, differential diagnosis is required.

Among these pathologies:

- phlyctenular keratoconjunctivitis
- squamous-cell carcinoma of the limbus
- pinguecula
- pseudo-pterygium
- lymphoma of the conjunctiva
- Bowen's disease or epithelioma
- nodular episcleritis
- epibulbar dermoid
- conjunctival papilloma

- **Phlyctenular keratoconjunctivitis** is a small circumscribed conjunctival neo-formation with a gel-like appearance and surrounded by twisted capillaries; it is associated with conjunctival hyperemia. The pathogenesis is linked to delayed hypersensitivity to foreign bacterial or food proteins. This pathology is generally localized, but in some cases can lead to new vessel formation in the cornea and successive surface opacity. It is common in infancy or childhood.

- **Squamous-cell carcinoma of the limbus** is a very rare pathology but its differential diagnosis may be difficult with respect to other pathologies of the limbus, including a pterygium. Like a pterygium, it would also appear to be the result of chronic exposure to UV radiation. The most common site is the infero-temporal zone of the limbus. The definitive diagnosis is obtained by histological examination *(Figures 10-1, 10-2)*.

- **Pinguecula** is a very common benign conjunctival pathology. It is round, raised to a greater or lesser degree, and whitish or yellowish in color. The most common site is the limbus. Fine twisted capillaries are often be found inside. From a histological point of view, pinguecula is the hyaline degeneration of the conjunctival connective tissue. It is normally asymptomatic but in some circumstances may show signs of inflammation with symptoms of burning, weeping, foreign body sensation. The differential diagnosis is against a pterygium Type I with a pinguecular appearance *(Figure 10-3)*.

- There may be some problems with the differential diagnosis between a **pterygium** and a **pseudo-pterygium**. The clinical appearances of pseudo-pterygium and pterygium are very similar but the exact pathogenesis of the two conditions is different. A pseudo-pterygium results from the repair of peripheral corneal ulcers or limbus inflammation of various origin (chemical, heat, microbiological, auto-immune). It can therefore be defined as the sectorial conjunctivalization of the corneal surface, and will appear in any corneal zone with no exceptions. It is not an evolutive lesion; however, if the damage of the limbus is extended around the entire circumference, a fibro-vascular layer may form which covers the entire cornea. It is not usually necessary to remove a pseudo-pterygium unless it damages the optical zone *(Figures 10-4, 10-5)*.

33

In some cases, it may be a complication resulting from the surgery of pterygium.

• **Lymphoma of the conjunctiva** is a very rare lesion that interests the inferior and nasal bulb conjunctiva. This is a salmon pink sub-conjunctival lesion which is poorly vascularized and almost flat. The definitive diagnosis is obtained histologically *(Figure 10-6)*.

• **Bowen's epithelioma** is a neoplastic proliferation of the limbus with local malignancy. It tends to infiltrate the cornea and the conjunctiva. The definitive diagnosis is histological *(Figures 10-7, 10-8)*.

• **The limbal dermoid** is a rare congenital pathology which appears as a round yellow-red neo-formation between the limbus and the edge of the cornea. There is no abnormal vascularization.

The preferred site for the dermoid is the infero-temporal sector *(Figure 10-9)*.

- **The papilloma** is a small active neo-formation the shape of a small cauliflower. It is highly vascular and bleeds easily. Compared to a pterygium differential diagnosis is easy but a certain diagnosis is histological. It is of viral origin *(Figure 10-10)*.

• **Nodular episcleritis** is an inflammation of the episclera and the over-lying conjunctiva; in the nodular forms it is localized. Young adult females are most affected and the pathology is observed as a bright red, almost flat nodule. It consists of twisted and injected conjunctival and episcleral capillary vessels. When it first appears, episcleritis is associated with pain but it disappears following several weeks' treatment with anti-inflammatory drugs. However, it tends to recur.

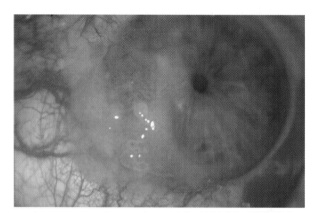

Figure 10-1. *Squamous-cell carcinoma of the limbus. The lesion is raised and irregular and invades the peripheral cornea. Degeneration of the epithelium is visible with squamous metaplasia.*

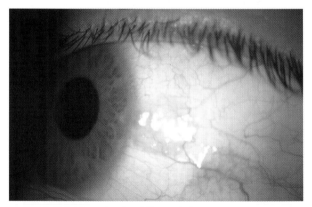

Figure 10-3. *Pinguecula. The differential diagnosis is consistent when compared against pterygium Type I with pinguecular appearance.*

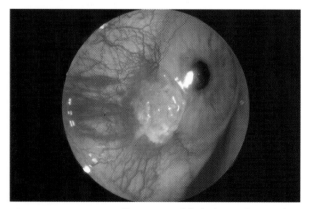

Figure 10-2. *Squamous-cell carcinoma of the limbus. In this case there is rich vascularization around the limbal lesion, the ectatic conjunctival capillaries are connected by anastomotic networks. Squamous metaplasia is clearly visible.*

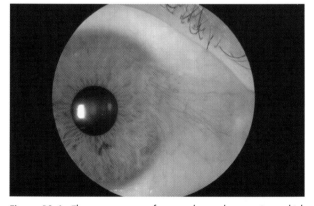

Figure 10-4. *The appearance of a nasal pseudo-pterygium which appeared following contact with slaked lime. It strongly resembles a pterygium even though it is in a slightly eccentric position with an oblique lesion progression. The clinical picture is stationary and surgery is not necessary.*

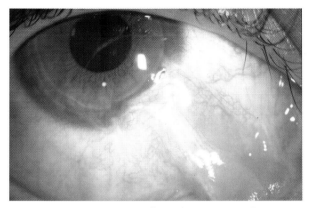

Figure 10-5. *The appearance of pseudo-pterygium with scar symblepharon resulting from burning with hydrochloric acid. The lesion is stable and only marginally invades the cornea. Surgery is necessary only if there are problems with eye movements.*

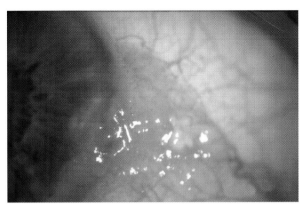

Figure 10-8. *Bowen's epithelioma. Gel-like appearance of the lesion. The infiltration of the cornea can be observed. There are some areas of squamous metaplasia visible as superficial whitish plates. Sometimes the differential diagnosis with "malignant" pterygia proves difficult, requiring histological examination of the tissue.*

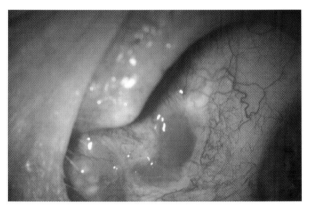

Figure 10-6. *The appearance of a primary lymphoma of the conjunctiva at the medial canthus. The B-cell lymphoma, with low grade malignancy appeared in three months. Elective treatment consists of localized radiotherapy.*

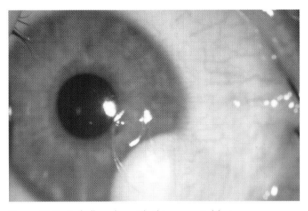

Figure 10-9. *Epibulbar dermoid. This congenital lesion appears as a pink, raised nodule, localized at the limbus.*
The lesion is not progressive and it is removed for aesthetic reasons only.

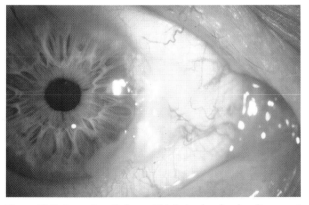

Figure 10-7. *Bowen's epithelioma. This lesion has local malignancy. It originates in the limbus and has slow progression and infiltration of the peripheral cornea. The appearance is one of a whitish lesion, raised with a gel-like appearance surrounded by a rich, fine network of newly-formed vessels.*

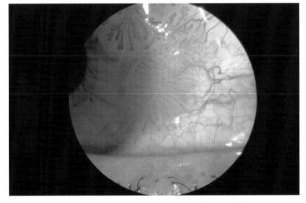

Figure 10-10. *Corneo-conjunctival papilloma. The neo-formation originates in the nasal limbus and invades the cornea. A feature of the lesion is the branching neo-vascularization. It is of viral origin.*

11

TREATMENT OF PTERYGIUM

In the past, a pterygium was considered to be a progressive pathology and surgery was always performed, even in the initial stages to block the growth on the cornea and reduce the risk of recurrence. This attitude has now changed and the decision to operate on a pterygium is based on the clinical picture: evolution on the cornea, progression, risk factors, symptoms and the patient's age.

However, even though there is general agreement on the indications, the most suitable forms of treatment and the surgical and para-surgical protocols to be used are the subject of debate and are still in the phase of clinical evaluation.

One method used to evaluate the efficacy of treatment for a pterygium is observation of the number of recurrences and complications. According to Hirst et al,[123] after treatment, one year follow-up is necessary. It has been observed that 97% of the recurrences appear in the 12-month period compared to only 50% in the first four months.

One-year follow-up is not sufficient for evaluation of the late complications, such as scleromalacia and episcleral granuloma following treatment with Mitomycin or beta-irradiation therapy, as these may appear even three years after treatment.

There are numerous options for treating pterygia; however, only a handful of techniques provide satisfactory and definitive results. Several other methods have not proved efficacious and have been abandoned.

Medical therapy, for example, has provided some results in the inflamed forms but proved to be completely useless in influencing the evolution of a pterygium. Therapy by physical means which

was the elective treatment of the Sixties, produced good results in the initial forms of pterygium but was a failure in the more advanced stages and was abandoned. Only photo-coagulation therapy with argon laser, in specially selected cases, and radiotherapy associated with surgery can be considered useful therapy by physical means in the recurrent forms.

Surgery is the most efficacious treatment for a pterygium, but it must only be performed when indicated. These indications are dependent on the clinical picture and the risk factors.

In the treatment of a pterygium, we can identify four therapeutic groups:

- **Medical treatment**
- **Treatment by chemical or physical means**
- **Surgical treatment**
- **Associated therapies**

MEDICAL TREATMENT

In past centuries, medical treatment involved the topical administration of galenic solutions to try to block the progression of a pterygium or to encourage scar formation following the surgical removal of the lesion. However, no medical therapy provided sufficient and long-lasting results.

In topical administration, cortisone has a certain degree of therapeutic efficacy in the inflamed forms of pterygia but it does not influence the subsequent clinical progression.

Perdriel's protocol (1958)[50] treated inflamed

pterygia or blocked the progression of the rapidly evolving forms by using four x 0.5-1.0 cc injections of hydrocortisone at 7/15-day intervals. The cortisone was injected directly into the body in correspondence to the head of the pterygium. The author reported a growth blockage in 50% of cases. In the past, sub-conjunctival administration of the enzyme hyaluronidase was also experimented but proved to be completely useless.[51]

In the treatment of the inflamed forms of pterygia and pinguecula, 1% indomethacin eyedrops provide therapeutic efficacy comparable to 1% dexamethasone eye-drops but with a lower degree of discomfort.[52]

The protocol involves six administrations per day for the first 3 days, followed by four administrations per day for a further 11 days.

Eye-drops of 1% indomethacin can therefore be considered the first line drug in the treatment of inflamed a pterygium and pinguecula or in those patients where topical cortisone is not indicated.

CHEMICAL/PHYSICAL THERAPY

Chemical caustication of pterygium and therapy by physical means have been used in the past to destroy the sub-conjunctival fibro-vascular tissue and the cells of a pterygium.

It was indicated for a small-size pterygium.

Results were disappointing and the majority of these techniques have been abandoned.

One specific indication, which lacks complications, is photo-coagulation of a pterygium with argon laser. The use of other laser sources is still in the experimental stage.

Radio-therapy with beta-emission combined with surgery is still being used.

Obsolete Techniques

• Caustication with carbolic acid
• Electrolysis
• Electro-coagulation
• Electric shock treatment
• Roentgen therapy
• Cryo-therapy

LASER TECHNIQUES

The treatment of pterygium with laser energy is a fairly recent development and is not widely used in clinical practice. It still requires long-term evaluation.

Photo-coagulation With Argon Laser

This is indicated in small stationary pterygium (Pterygium Type I) and is an alternative technique to straightforward excision surgery. The treatment is indicated in patients that require the operation for aesthetic reasons or in patients who refuse surgery. Treatment of a pterygium with argon laser is also indicated in ametropic patients with intolerance to contact lenses. In clinical experience, the blue/green light of the argon laser can be used to treat primary pterygia.[53,54,55] The heat produced by the argon laser photo-coagulates the blood vessel in the head and body of pterygium and retracts the sub-conjunctival fibrovascular tissue. The final effect is bleaching and flattening of the tissue with regression of the lesion.

Regression of pterygia is progressive in the three months following treatment and persists in time. No long term findings are available, but according to Caldwell, recurrences are reduced to approximately 1% of cases following this treatment.[124]

Technique

Treatment may be performed in a single session or in 2-3 sessions at 5/10-day intervals. Topical anesthesia is sufficient and the treatment is performed without optical devices.

The blue/green or green wavelength of the argon laser can be used.

The use of fluorescein will increase the laser's thermal effect in the treatment zone, limiting damage to the surrounding conjunctiva. Staining with fluorescein can be performed with a paper tip normally used in tonometry or with a triangular sponge soaked in a solution of fluorescein as normally used for fluorangiography.

In technical terms, photo-coagulation with argon laser can be split into two separate phases.

Phase 1 (Photo-coagulation of the vessels)

Direct photo-coagulation of the larger vessels for the entire length of the body to the apex with small spots (100 microns) and an appropriate power level (normally 400-600 mW or 200-300 mW with fluorescein); exposure time of 0.1-0.2 seconds.

The impact must produce the immediate occlusion of the vascular lumen with evident whitening of the impact site.

Photo-coagulation must be performed on all major vessels and should be extended to include the peripheral vessels that define the upper and lower limits of the body of pterygium.

Phase 2 (Thermal retraction)

Spots of larger diameter (200-300 microns) and lower power levels are used (150-300 mW or 100-200 mW with fluorescein); exposure time of 0.5 seconds. In order to avoid burning the conjunctiva excessively (observed as a hole with a black outline) the laser beam must be defocussed in depth.

This will concentrate the thermal effect on the sub-conjunctival tissue instead of on the mucosa, and the thermal effect on this layer appears as contraction of the tissue at the impact site.

Post-operative course

Redness, burning and foreign body sensation may be observed in the 24-48 hours following treatment; pain is rare.

Following each treatment session, topical cortisone (Clobetasone Butyrate, 0.1% Fluormetholone) or 0.1-0.5% indomethacin, three times a day for one week, is an efficacious treatment to control the mild inflammation and irritation.

Photo-coagulation With Yag Laser

If the Yag-laser is used in the free-running, thermal mode, with power levels of 0.6-0.8 mJ, the heat effects are superimposable to the argon laser.[53] There are no reports on the use of the mechanical Yag-laser.

Photoablation With Excimer Laser

In the past, in order to prevent the re-appearance of pterygium, to produce a smooth, even corneal surface was considered to be an essential step following surgery. For this purpose, superficial keratectomies were performed using instruments that were specially designed for scraping and cleaning the cornea; drills with diamond bits, flesh-stripping spatulas etc.

Seiler[56] was the first to suggest using the excimer laser for this purpose. The excimer laser emits a coherent light beam corresponding to the UV spectrum (193 nm). This produces extremely precise photoablation, both in depth and extension. The technique involves a keratectomy with excimer laser of the infiltrated irregular surface following the excision of the head of pterygium. For laser keratectomy, viscous substances based on methyl-cellulose or sodium hyaluronate are used to fill the spaces between the residual tissue to be ablated (photo-therapeutic keratectomy or PTK).

The operation ends with the repair of the scleral surface and plastic surgery of the conjunctiva, even when the treatment has been associated with techniques of scleral baring, with or without Mitomicin C.[57,58]

The surface treated with the excimer laser is very smooth, even and, depending on the depth of the keratectomy, transparent.

Results

Poor results have been reported for the treatment with excimer laser with recurrences observed in 80-90% of cases one year after treatment.[56,57,58,125] Irregular post-operative astigmatism that has proved difficult to treat has also been reported.

There is little experience in the photo-therapeutic treatment (PTK) of the optical zone following the removal of advanced pterygium.

Frequently, following successful surgery, there may be an irregular optical zone with superficial opacity of the stroma which will cause a marked reduction in vision.

Laser treatment of the optical zone for therapeutic reasons, while being a commonly used method for many pathologies, in pterygia must still be considered experimental. In the future, it may prove to be a valid alternative to lamellar keratoplasty.

However, at this stage, there is also the possibility that excimer laser treatment, even when distant from the limbus and the peripheral cornea, may stimulate biological mechanisms that can encourage a recurrence or activate a stationary pterygium.

RADIOTHERAPY OF PTERYGIA

High energy radiation application to treat pterygia has been used for more than 50 years. X-rays were the first to be used with the epi-bulbar technique, but the side effects on the globe were frequent and serious (radiation cataracts, retinopathies). As a result, this practice was abandoned.

Beta-therapy using beta-emission radioactive substances was proposed by Burnham and Reudmann in 1941 and is still being used today.

Beta-Therapy

Therapy with beta radiation is performed using beta-emission radioactive substances which act when in close contact with the tissue to be treated. The penetration of the effect of this type of radiation is limited to a few millimeters; it produces arteriolar obliteration and a block of connective tissue and fibroblast proliferation.

The beta-emission radioactive substances used in the treatment of pterygium are Strontium-90 (Sr-90), Radium D + E and Ruthenium 106 (Ru106).[59]

Ruthenium 106 (Ru106)

A Ruthenium 106 (Ru106) plate is not commonly used.

The plate is sutured in the treatment site and left in situ for 2-3 hours until the emission levels reach approximately 2000 cGy.

Only a handful of cases have been treated with Ruthenium and numerous cases of recurrences have been reported, in addition to constant corneal haze that appears precociously but which regresses over the weeks that follow.

Strontium-90 (Sr-90)

This is the most common beta-emission substance used in the treatment of pterygia and in other neoplasms of the eye surface. It has a half-life of 28 years and decomposes to yttrium 90 which has a half-life of 64 hours. It does not emit gamma radiation and its effect does not exceed 2 mm depth.

The energy dosing and the application are performed by a radiotherapist.

Beta-therapy is measured in Gray (Gy).

1 Gy = 100 cGy = 100 rad of exposure
1 rep = Roentgen equivalent physical
1 rep = 1.08 rad = 1.08 cGy
1 Gy = 92.6 rep
1 sievert (sv) = 100 rem (absorbed dose)

Technique

Radiotherapy of a pterygium is always associated with the surgical technique of scleral baring. The radioactive applicator is placed in contact with the bare sclera.

When a superficial treatment is required, not penetrating more than 1 mm in depth, or when the damage of the sclera must be limited, two soft hydrophilic contact lenses (70% hydrophilic) of 0.5 mm thickness each are applied. These lenses will restrict the penetration of the beta radiation to within 1 mm depth.[60]

The applicator is placed at the limbus in three adjacent points; alternately the dose is applied by the emitter through a circular movement around the limbus.[67]

The dose may be single or split over the following few days but never four days from surgery.

There are a number of treatment protocols and dosing schedules available. Which one is chosen is the responsibility of the radiotherapist[61] (see table below). The total dose administered lies between 1000 cGy and 7000 cGy, but is generally 5000 cGy.[62] The total dose varies if the dose is single or multiple.

For single doses, 1000-2000 cGy are generally applied; in split doses 800 cGy per dose is normal and for 3-6 weeks, or alternately four doses of 1296 cGy (three minutes of application) at 8-day intervals.[62,63,64,65]

Another protocol involves a single dose of 2000-3000 cGy applied to the bare sclera during the operation or four days later.[61,65,66]

A Study Group for pterygium based in Florida recommends an intraoperative dose of 2000-6000 cGy. A very low incidence of recurrences is reported.[67]

PROTOCOLS FOR THE SINGLE DOSE OF SR90		
Dose	**Application**	**Author**
2000-3000 cGy	Intraoperative	Beyer
2000-3000 cGy	Four days later	Beyer
2000-6000 cGy	Intraoperative	North Florida Study Group
1800-2200 cGy	2-48 hours	Bahrassa
1000-2000 cGy	Intraoperative	Neal

PROTOCOLS FOR SPLIT DOSES OF SR90			
Dose	**No. doses**	**Interval**	**Author**
800 cGy	3-6	7 days	Wilder
1296 cGy	4	8 days	Campbell
1080 cGy	3	7 days	De Keizer
500 cGy	4	1 day	Hayasaka
1000 cGy	6	7 days	Paryani
1500 cGy	2	1-48 hours	Bhatti

Post-operative course

Reactive conjunctivitis with hyperemia, burning and foreign body sensation are always observed in the post-operative clinical course. These symptoms may persist for several weeks.

At the slit lamp, the conjunctiva is reddened around the treated sclera, there is mild catarrhal secretion and sloughing of the conjunctival epithelium and the cornea are often observed.

Post-operative treatment consists of topical cortisone or Nsaids (Indomethacin - diclofenac) 3-4 times a day, starting on the day of treatment and continued for at least 7-10 days after treatment.

Complications with beta therapy

Early or late complications can be observed even years after treatment.

• The epithelial defects of the cornea and the paralimbal zones of corneal and scleral thinning are the earliest complications of beta-therapy and may appear within 2-3 weeks from treatment. These complications are usually moderate but in some cases may lead to the formation of evident limbal ulcers.[61, 71] The post-operative course is generally benign and the ulcers tend to heal spontaneously in a matter of weeks.

• Radionecrosis of the cornea and the sclera is the most serious complication. It appears initially as a corneal, scleral or mixed ulcer, accompanied by a violent inflammatory reaction over the entire globe surface and the anterior segment.[72] The symptoms are very obvious and can be reduced with topical steroid or NSAID therapy. Healing of these areas leads to scleromalacia and/or secondary calcification. Scleral necrosis and scleritis are generally of late onset, from 1-2 months to years after treatment.[71,73,74,76]

• Episcleral granulomas are rare and along with the calcific plates produce an excellent medium for the growth of saprophytic, pathogenic and fungal germs *(Figure 11-1)*.

• Infections and endophthalmitis have been observed following the removal of episcleral granulomas and calcific plates.[72] These infections

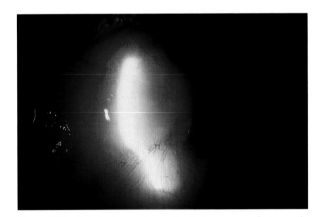

Figure 11-1. *Episcleral granuloma. The lesion appeared six months following the application of Sr-90 to treat a recurrent pterygium. Removal is always necessary and must be completed under local and systemic antibiotic prophylaxis. Sometimes a thinned scleral area remains.*

are generally caused by Streptococci and Pseudomonas aeruginosa (bacteria), and Aspergillus and Fusarium (mycetes). The removal of a granuloma or calcific plate must be performed under conditions of maximum sterility with pre- and post-operative antibiotic prophylaxis.

- Areas of scleromalacia are frequently observed and include the areas of thinning observed in 5-13% of treated patients and the classical scleramalacia itself.[70]

- A cataract is rare and may appear several years later.[59]

- Ptosis (damage to the levator muscle) and exodeviation (damage to the medial rectus muscle) are rarely observed.

- Scar symblepharon has been reported following high dose beta therapy.

- Posterior scleritis has been reported in some rare cases. This is a very serious complication that is difficult to diagnose and treat.

- Corneal scarring has been observed in about 0.3% of cases.[70]

Results

The results reported in the literature are positive and there is a considerable reduction in the recurrences to between 1.7-14%.[64,61,60,69,70]

Conclusions

Beta therapy with Strontium 90 (Sr-90) contributes to reducing the incidence of the recurrences relapses. However, due to the non-selective action of the beta radiation, the globe may be subject to delayed repair processes and serious complications.

The recurrences and the complications would appear to be directly proportional to the total dose of radiation applied, and for equal doses, splitting the applications reduces the complications and the side effects.

TABLE OF THE RESULTS REPORTED IN THE LITERATURE					
Dose Sr-90	No. appl.	No. patients	Follow-up	% Relapses	Author
2500 cGy	2	256	N.R.	3.6	Lentino
800-1000 cGy	3	1300	3 months	1.7	Van Den Brenk
700-800 cGy	4	485	N.R.	4.3	Alaniz-Calamino
900-1000 cGy	3	37	6-40 months	0	De Keizer
600 cGy	3	135	N.R.	7.4	Morseline
800 cGy	3	258	6-24 months	12.8	Wilder
3240 cGy	1	200	1-27 months	0.5	Walter
1000 cGy	6	825	1-8 years	1.7	Paryani
2200 cGy	1	585	10 years	12	MacKenzie
1800-2200 cGy	1	83	4-8 years	5	Bahrassa
1000 cGy	3	272	N.R.	11.8	Cooper

12
SURGERY OF PTERYGIUM

Informing the patient on the surgical objectives and the possible results is a fundamental part of treatment.

The information must also include the percentage success rate of the operation, with a full explanation that, due to the biological nature of a pterygium, a recurrence is possible and that this may be more serious than the initial condition.

Surgery is the elective treatment, for primary and recurrent pterygium and the numerous techniques available range from simple surgical removal to the more complex techniques with mucous membrane grafts and keratoplasty.

As we will see, the choice of technique depends on the final objective and the severity of the clinical picture.

INDICATIONS AND OBJECTIVES OF SURGERY

Excisional surgery for aesthetic reasons is indicated for a small stationary Type I pterygium that only marginally involves the cornea and which does not reduce vision or cause irritation. It is often requested by the patient.

The objective of surgery is to remove the head of pterygium and repair of the conjunctiva simply by sealing the wound margins. When the operation is performed correctly, recurrences are rare and the aesthetic result is excellent.

In the more advanced pterygium Type II, surgery is indicated particularly for the progressive forms - the advanced lesions that tend to reach and

invade the optical zone. Surgery has a two-fold objective: it must remove the lesion and prevent the pathology from re-appearing. In this group of patients, simple removal is not indicated because of the high risk of recurrences that occur in up to 80% of all cases.

In pterygium Type III where the optical zone has already been invaded, surgery is always necessary to restore sight. Surgery must primarily aim for: the removal of pterygium from the cornea, the reduction of the recurrences, the treatment of the optical zone, and in many cases, the repair of the conjunctiva because of the large resections necessary to eliminate the subconjunctival fibro-vascular proliferation.

Objectives of Surgery

- **Pterygium Type I:** removal of a pterygium for aesthetic reasons, leaving a smooth, even peripheral corneal surface, particularly in the event the patient wears contact lenses and the pterygium has created intolerance. Sealing and suturing of the conjunctiva.

- **Pterygium Type II:** Removal to prevent progression of a pterygium towards the optical zone and reduction in the number of recurrences. Repair of the conjunctival tissue loss.

- **Pterygium Type III:** removal of the pterygium and prevention of the recurrences with transparency of the corneal optical zone restored. Repair of the conjunctival loss and correction of the fibrous growths of the conjunctival flap.

CLASSIFICATION OF THE PTERYGIUM OPERATIONS

The operations for a pterygium can be classed on the basis of the objectives:

1. Simple surgical removal (Pterygium Type I)

2. Barrier surgery to prevent recurrences (Pterygium Type II)

3. Treatment of the optical zone (Pterygium Type III)

4. Surgery for conjunctival re-construction (Pterygium Type II and III).

1. Simple Surgical Removal

This form of surgery removes small stationary pterygia (Type I). The techniques are simple and are restricted to the removal of the head from the limbus and from the peripheral cornea, and removal of the small body of the pterygium. Repair of the conjunctiva is simple: the two edges of the wound are sealed and the conjunctival edges are sutured.

- **Indications:** Stationary Pterygium Type I

- **Objectives:** removal of the lesion and aesthetically acceptable results

2. Barrier Surgery to Prevent Relapses

This is indicated in the treatment of a primary or recurrent pterygium that is actively progressing towards the corneal optical zone.

This technique actually creates a mechanical or biological barrier at the limbus against the progression of the recurrent pterygium. The barrier is created with mucosal or corneal tissue grafts, at the limbus or peripheral cornea respectively, or by inhibiting fibroblastic mitosis with anti-tumor drugs or radiation therapy applied to the bare sclera following removal of pterygium.

Subdivisions of this group are:

1. Free autologous graft of conjunctival tissue
2. Peripheral lamellar keratoplasty
3. Operations of scleral baring and treatment with anti-tumor drugs or radiation therapy

4. Grafts of a colonized biological substrate with autologous limbal stem cells (prospects for the future).

Indications: primary or recurrent pterygium Type II that show clinical signs of progression towards the optical zone.

Objectives: removal of the lesion and barrier surgery against recurrences.

The table shows the percentage recurrences reported by some authors with the various barrier techniques.

Operation	% Recurr.	Author	Year
Conjunctival Autologous graft	5.3%	Kenyon	1985
»	20%	Vaniscotte	1986
»	21%	Lewallen	1989
»	13.3%	Ferentini	1992
»	16%	Figueredo	1997
Lamellar keratoplasty	3%	Laughrea	1986
»	7.7%	Busin	1986
»	17.6%	Vaniscotte	1986
Bare sclera + Mito C	5%	Frucht-Pery	1994
»	6.6%	Mastropasqua	1994
»	5.75%	Helal	1996
Bare sclera + Betatherapy	5%	Bahrassa	1983
»	12%	Mackenzie	1991
»	0.5%	Walter	1994

3. Treatment of the Optical Zone

This form of surgery is indicated for the treatment of opacities created by a pterygium in the optical zone, considered to be the distinguishing feature of Pterygium Type III.

The objective of this type of surgery is to create a regular, transparent cornea following the removal of the head and the infiltrated cornea.

The treatment of the optical zone can be performed when the pterygium is being removed or alternately in a subsequent operation, when there is no risk of recurrence.

The therapeutic possibilities are:

1. lamellar keratoplasty manual, circular, central, wide or total

2. lamellar keratoplasty simple mechanized or laser assisted

3. photo-reactive keratectomy with excimer laser (PTK)

4. penetrating keratoplasty

Indications: advanced primary or relapsed pterygium with the optical zone compromised (Pterygium Type III).

Objectives: to restore transparency and regularity of the corneal optical zone.

4. Surgery for Conjunctival Re-construction

This group includes the operations with mucosal tissue grafts and plastic surgery of the conjunctiva to repair the scleral surface exposed by the removal of the body.

The type of conjunctival repair depends on the extension of the surface to be covered, the abundance of sub-conjunctival fibrous tissue and concomitant oculo-motory and conjunctival complications (symblepharon, adduction deficit, epiphora, enophthalmos).

The treatment possibilities are:

• free autologous conjunctival graft

• plastic surgery of the conjunctiva by stretching and torsion

• free graft of amniotic membrane

• free graft of buccal mucosa.

Indications: recurrent pterygium Type II and Type III with abundant sub-conjunctival fibrovascular proliferation.

Objectives: reconstruction of the conjunctival flap.

13

SURGICAL TECHNIQUE

This section will describe the important surgical steps of all the operations used in the pterygium and the principal variations used when removing the head and the body of the lesion.

The first, more general part is dedicated to the types of anesthesia used in pterygium surgery.

The successive chapters will cover the surgical techniques for the treatment of progressive and advanced pterygia: the techniques of lamellar keratoplasty, the surgery used to repair the conjunctiva and the techniques of sclera baring with protocols that include treatment with mitomycin.

GENERAL SECTION

Anesthesia

Topical anesthesia is used when the removal involves small Type I pterygia.

The most efficacious anesthetic agents that produce good anesthesia are oxybupivacaine, 2-4% Lidocaine instilled 4 times in the 10-20 minutes before surgery begins.

In the more advanced forms of pterygia pterygium, Types II and III, infiltration anesthesia is advisable using 2-4% Lidocaine, 10% Ropivacaine hydrochloride. During infiltration, the anesthetic agent is injected under the body of the pterygium. Diffusion throughout the tissue is assisted by massaging the eye with a sponge tip or a spatula. Because of the biological nature of the fibrous tissue found in pterygium, spontaneous diffusion of all anesthetic agents is very poor.

Peribulbar or retrobulbar anesthesia, in addition to producing excellent analgesia, also permits good control of the globe motility which is very important in lamellar keratoplasty.

General anesthesia is indicated in cases of lamellar keratoplasty of the optical zone and when the surgeon is learning this surgical technique.

Removal of Pterygium

Removal of pterygium is a surgical step common to all techniques.

Some steps can be identified:

1. Detachment of the head. This is possible using one of two methods: avulsing or the progressive dissection of the head using a sharp instrument.

Avulsing is performed by catching the head of the pterygium for its full depth with toothed conjunctival forceps, and pulling the tissue upwards to detach it from the underlying corneal adhesions. In small-sized pterygia, and in the primary forms in general, avulsion is fairly simple and consents the complete removal of the head, leaving an underlying surface that is smooth and very regular. In the more extended forms of pterygium and in the recurrent forms, where there is greater corneal infiltration, avulsing proves to be more difficult and the dissection technique is preferable or alternately the pterygium can be removed by scissors or other sharp instruments.

The **dissection** can be performed using scissors or other sharp blade instruments - disc or rectangular spatula for example. The head of the pterygium is caught and pulled using conjunctival forceps, in the same way as avulsing. The cutting instrument is positioned tangentially at the base of the lesion and the head is detached from the underlying adhesions. During this maneuver, a keratectomy of the superficial stromal layers is necessary and should be performed as deep as the more transparent layers of the cornea. It is important that the keratectomy is performed on the same plane to avoid irregularities that may lead to recurrences or may cause irregular astigmatism. The detachment of the head and its dissection must extend beyond the surgical limbus to reach the initial part of the body *(Figures 13-1, 13-2)*.

2. Excision of the body of the pterygium.

In the small pterygium, the body progressively invades the healthy conjunctiva and excision must follow detachment of the surrounding conjunctiva. The detachment is performed with blunt conjunctival scissors in order to avoid fissures and damage to the healthy conjunctiva; it must also be sufficiently wide to facilitate tension-free sealing and suturing of the edges when the conjunctiva is being repaired.

Excision of pterygium must include the head detached from the cornea and the body. It is not necessary to remove the surrounding healthy conjunctiva to avoid creating difficulties in the subsequent plastic surgery repairs.

The excision can be triangular *(Figure 13-3)*, by means of two cuts that extend just beyond the edge of the body to reach the internal canthus; alternately, it can be square or rectangular with cuts parallel to the body, and a third cut perpendicular to these.

In the cases of more advanced pterygia, where the body is hypertrophic and there is massive sub-conjunctival fibrosis, excision may damage the tendon of the medial rectus muscle. In order to avoid this unpleasant complication, we suggest positioning a strabismus hook under the tendon *(Figure 13-4)* to permit direct visualization. The shape of the excision conditions the subsequent plastic surgery technique to repair the conjunctiva.

Ziegler's technique differs from the other excision techniques as it allows the selective removal of sub-conjunctival fibro-vascular tissue, avoiding involvement of the conjunctival mucous flap. The technique involves the complete detachment of the body from the underlying sclera, as far as the semilunar fold, hemostasis of the episclera and the removal of fibrovascular fragments. The body of the pterygium is pulled upwards by the surgeon's assistant, using two forceps or two 8/0 silk threads.

The surgeon, with fine forceps and pointed scissors, progressively removes the sub-conjunctival tissue, avoiding damage to the superficial conjunctival layer.

The removal must be performed very carefully and must extend as far as the semilunar fold. Fissures or lacerations of the conjunctiva can annul the benefits of this technique because any damaged conjunctiva must be removed. Following removal of the fibrovascular tissue, the conjunctiva appears thin and transparent. The biggest advantage of this technique is that the conjunctival tissue is preserved, a useful factor if large surfaces have to be repaired as plastic surgery with mucosal tissue grafts can be avoided.

When the head and body of pterygium have been removed, some fibrous tissue usually remains at the limbus or in the peripheral cornea. This should be removed with a dry sponge tip or scraped away using a blunt instrument

During the operation, the surface of the sclera may bleed easily because of the fibrovascular tissue present *(Figure 13-5)*. Hemostasis and removal of this tissue are necessary in order to obtain a white, blood-free scleral surface.

Hemostasis must be performed gently and patiently; all the various systems available can be used: heat-cauterization, diathermy, low intensity radio-frequency or simply a spatula heated over a flame.

The larger fragments of episcleral tissue can be removed with forceps and Vannas scissors. When the scleral surface appears to be blood-free and cleaned of episcleral tissue, the surgeon can proceed to the next surgical stage *(Figure 13-6)*.

3. Repair of the conjunctiva.
This surgical step concludes the pterygium operations and is very important for the final aesthetic outcome.

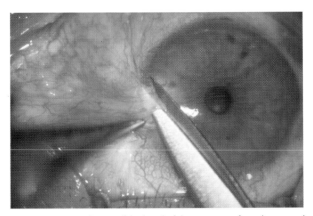

Figure 13-1. *Detachment of the head of the pterygium from the corneal insertion using scissors. The head is placed under slight tension with forceps and cut with scissors placed tangential to the corneal surface. Removing the head of the pterygium with scissors leaves numerous tissue fragments which will have to be removed at a later stage.*

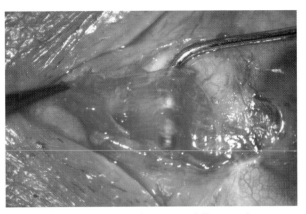

Figure 13-4. *Excision of the sub-conjunctival fibro-vascular tissue. In order to avoid damaging the tendon of the medial rectus muscle, a strabismus needle is inserted under the tendon and is constantly kept in view.*

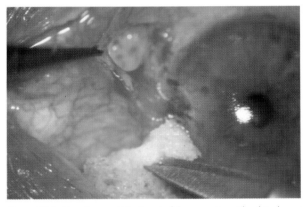

Figure 13-2. *Detachment of the head of the pterygium. The detachment of the head should involve both the corneal surface and the collarette at the limbus and proceed in the body of the lesion.*

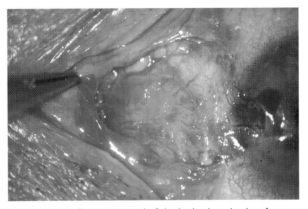

Figure 13-5. *Following removal of the body, the scleral surface appears to be bleeding and covered in fibro-vascular tissue. The conjunctiva is pushed back towards the semilunar fold and the scleral surface can be coagulated.*

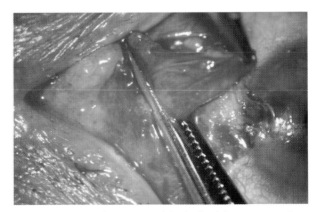

Figure 13-3. *Triangular excision of the body of the pterygium. Once the head has been eliminated, along with the body of the pterygium, the sub-conjunctival fibro-vascular tissue is isolated and removed, preferable in one piece, as far as the semilunar fold.*

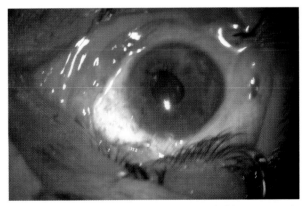

Figure 13-6. *The operating field following removal of the pterigium, the fibro-vascular tissue is cleaned and the episcleral vessels are coagulated.*

In Pterygium Type I, the repair is simply a question of sealing the conjunctival margins and suturing. In the cases where the removal of conjunctiva is more extensive, this technique is not sufficient and the surgeon must perform plastic surgery involving stretching or the addition of free grafts of mucosal tissue.

Simple sealing. This is the simplest method for covering small surfaces, particularly if they are triangular. Repair of larger areas is more difficult with this technique as it creates excessive traction on the conjunctiva which will tend to escape from the joining line and produce separation of the margins and exposure of the sclera.

The aesthetic result in these cases is not satisfactory because the exposed sclera heals due to secondary intention.

The conjunctiva surrounding the surface to be covered is detached with scissors and mobilized to bring the edges together without tension being created; the edges are sutured with monofilament 8/0 silk or 7/0-8/0 vicryl suture.

A useful hint is to pass the needle through the superficial layers of the scleral to release the tension and increase the adhesion of the conjunctiva to the underlying plane. *(Drawings 13-1, 13-2, 13-3).*

When the conjunctival edges are brought together under excessive tension, it is better to repair the wound by sliding as this will avoid creating an anti-aesthetic conjunctival scar *(Figure 13-7).*

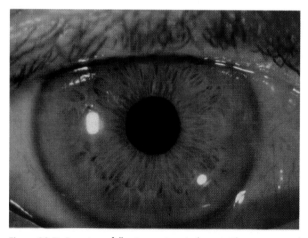

Figure 13-7. *Scar tissue following conjunctival repair. The traction used to close the conjunctival flaps was excessive, and resulted in unaesthetic scarring.*

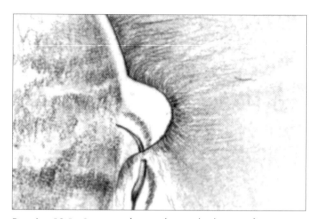

Drawing 13-1. *Conjunctival repair by simple closure. After removing the head and the small body, and after having coagulated the sclera, the repair of the small scleral surface occurs simply by closing the conjunctival edges. The drawing shows the needle pass through the lower edge of the conjunctiva which must be detached from the underlying episcleral adhesions so that it is more mobile.*

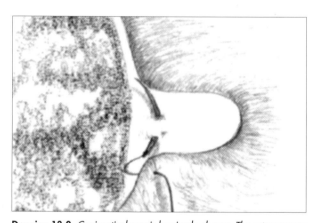

Drawing 13-2. *Conjunctival repair by simple closure. The suture passes through the superficial layers of the sclera about 2 mm from the limbus prior to passing through the superior edge of the conjunctiva. This technical detail is particularly useful for a number of reasons; it discharges the tension onto a fixed point, it increases the adhesion of the conjunctiva and the attachment in the post-operative. It also allows the surgeon to distance the conjunctival edge from the limbus, so the corneal re-epithelialization is encouraged instead of the conjunctival.*

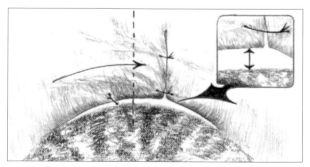

Drawing 13-3. *The conjunctival edges must be sutured about 2 mm from the limbus, decentered with respect to the median line so that the scarring occurs in a different position to where the pterygium was located (transposition of the scar line).*

14

LAMELLAR KERATOPLASTY IN PTERYGIUM SURGERY

HISTORY

The history of lamellar keratoplasty began at the beginning of this century with Fuchs (1911). He communicated the initial results with his technique in pathologies of the peripheral cornea; pterygia were excluded from the indications.

Terson (1913) included it among the indications for lamellar keratoplasty and reported therapeutic efficacy in recurrent or highly evolved pterygia.

Contrary to the authors that preceded him, Magitot (1916) suggested autologous lamellar keratoplasty in pterygium; removal of a flap in the superior quadrant of the cornea and grafting to the corneal site where the pterygium had been removed with a circular keratectomy. The results of the autologous lamellar keratoplasty were affected by numerous infective and trophic complications of the graft and this explains the poor dissemination of this technique which has been abandoned for many decades.

In the fifties, thanks to the French school of Paufique, homologous lamellar keratoplasty was adopted as the elective technique for many pathologies of the peripheral cornea, including a pterygium.

In Italy, since the sixties, Rama's school made an important contribution to the use of lamellar keratoplasty for the treatment of many pathologies of the eye surface and in the pterygium is considered to be the most suitable lamellar technique for each individual clinical picture.

INDICATIONS AND OBJECTIVES

For various reasons, lamellar keratoplasty (LK) is an important technique in the treatment of evolved pterygium Type III with compromised optical zone and in pterygium Type II with a progressive evolution. The objectives of lamellar keratoplasty are normally as follows:

- **Replacement of the tissue:** this is necessary when a deep extended keratectomy is performed in a pterygium excision.

- **Barrier:** theoretically, a compact tissue constitutes a valid barrier against recurrence of pterygium and this has been confirmed by the clinical results and the observation that the vessels from the limbus tend to surround the corneal graft, rather than penetrate to the inside or invade the surfaces.

- **Therapeutic:** the therapeutic effect of a corneal graft is not well-known and is possibly explained through a number of different mechanisms; a probable trophic effect and the inhibition of angiogenesis, connected to the protein degeneration of the corneal fibers infiltrated by the pterygium.

- **Optical:** the optical objective of lamellar keratoplasty is considered necessary when the extension of the pterygium directly or indirectly invades the optical zone of the cornea. The reduction in vision in pterygium Type II is caused by induced irregular astigmatism or through alterations of the lacrimal film surrounding the head of the lesion. In Pterygium Type III, there is a marked reduction in vision produced by the invasion of the optical zone. Lamellar keratoplasty, in a variety of ways, restores transparency to the optical zone and improves the astigmatism induced to the peripheral cornea and in the optical zone with improvements in sight. Generally speaking, the improvement of vision is not predictable due to the possible alterations with the manual creation of the interface. We would hope that in the future, the treatment of the optical zone in pterygium Type III will involve the use of the latest generation of microkeratome or excimer laser to perform the central keratectomy and to improve the surfaces of the interface.

- **Aesthetic:** even though it is not the primary treatment objective, the aesthetic result of lamellar keratoplasty greatly satisfies the patients.

THE SHAPE OF THE FLAP IN LAMELLAR KERATOPLASTY

The shape of the lamellar keratoplasty depends on the clinical characteristics of pterygium and on its extension on the cornea.

The peripheral half-moon graft is the most effective technique in the treatment of pterygium Type II (Both progressive and recurrent); the graft creates an important barrier effect against recurrences and an excellent aesthetic and optical result. In pterygium Type III, which has a compromised optical zone, the graft must be circular and be of sufficient diameter to include the entire optical zone. With the peripheral edge, it must reach the limbal site of the pterygium.

The peripheral half-moon and the large diameter circular graft represent the most popular shapes of LK in surgery of pterygium; in some special cases, during this specific operation or in a subsequent one, grafts with different shapes allow very extensive pterygia to be operated or alternately complications of the lamellar keratoplasty itself to be treated.

In choosing the shape and diameter of the graft, several factors must be taken into account:

- In the peripheral half-moon lamellar keratoplasty, the optical zone should not be invaded by with the edge of the graft;

- A diameter of 6 mm is the minimum optical zone which will avoid secondary disturbances of vision; however, in elderly patients, satisfactory results can be obtained with smaller optical zones.

- In the central circular keratoplasty, the diameter of the flap must not be less than the diameter of the optical zone with the over-sizing lying between 0.1 - 0.5 mm.

- In large or total keratoplasty, the flap diameter must be at least 11 mm.

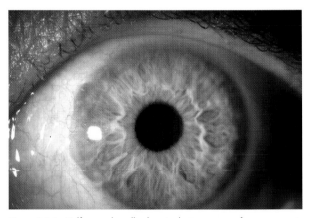

Figure 14-1. *Half-moon lamellar keratoplasty one year from surgery. In this Figure the therapeutic result of the operation and the excellent aesthetic result are clearly visible. The half-moon flap is perfectly transparent and the underlying iris tissue is clearly visible. The aesthetic result on the cornea would appear to be very good, while in the conjunctiva, a scarred area can be observed caused by an excessively tight conjunctival suture.*

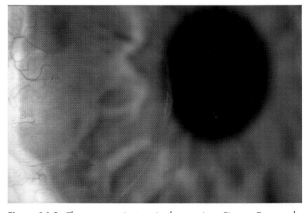

Figure 14-2. *The same patient as in the previous Figure. Even under greater magnification, the interface between the flap and the underlying cornea cannot be identified.*

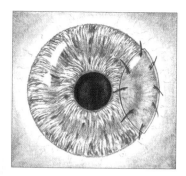

Drawing 14-1. *Peripheral half-moon graft.*
This is the simplest form and the most commonly used in a pterygium Type II. The radius of curvature of the flap is in relation to how peripheral the keratectomy is and its extension. The convexity faces the cornea and the radius of curvature is inversely proportional to the diameter of the trephine used for the preparation. The half-moon must respect an optical zone of at least 6 mm.

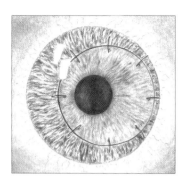

Drawing 14-4. *Decentered circular graft.*
The graft must be large enough to cover at least 6 mm of optical zone; however the nasal edge must reach the limbus at the site of the pterygium.

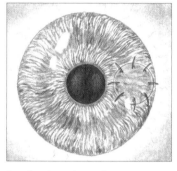

Drawing 14-2. *Peripheral circular graft.*
This is a circular flap of maximum diameter 5-6 mm. This shape is an alternative to the peripheral half-moon. The diameter is chosen on the basis that the corneal convexity has to exclude the optical zone while the limbal convexity must correspond to the limbal site of the pterygium.

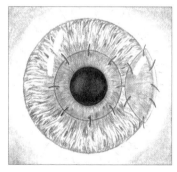

Drawing 14-5. *Association of flaps.*
The peripheral half-moon graft attempts to block the recurrence by means of a mechanical barrier. The central circular 6 mm graft aims to restore transparency and smoothness to the optic zone. The central optic LK can be performed at a later stage than the peripheral LK, when we have reached the therapeutic objective of the first operation: the absence of a recurrence.

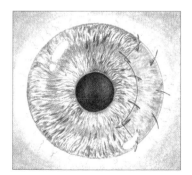

Drawing 14-3. *Half-washer peripheral graft.*
This shape is difficult to produce due to the angles between the flap and the cornea, and has not demonstrated any specific advantages over the half-moon with the exception of extending the optical zone. The choice of this graft is justified in pterygia with large extension of the collarette to the limbus and poor corneal extension.

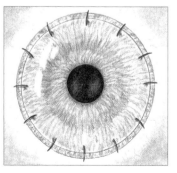

Drawing 14-6. *Large circular graft.*
This is the recommended shape for pterygium Type III that invades the pupil. The diameter of the flap lies between 9.1 mm and 12.1 mm.

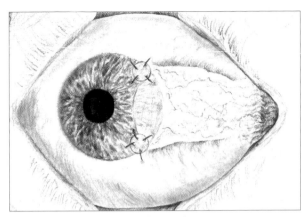

Drawing 14-7. *Small diameter patchwork shapes.*
In the cases where, following peripheral lamellar keratoplasty, a ptery-
gium tends to recur at the extremity of the graft, it is possible to graft
two small flaps at the extremity of the previous half-moon graft.

• In the decentered circular form, the diameter of the graft must cover a minimal optical zone of 6 mm and the nasal edge of the graft must correspond to the limbus.

DEPTH OF THE KERATECTOMY AND THICKNESS OF THE GRAFT

A pterygium is included among the pathologies of the eye surface and its natural evolution is to invade the corneal stroma. The depth of the invasion of the stroma lies at around 150 - 250 microns, but in some cases of repeatedly recurrent pterygia, the stromal opacities can involve up to 50% of the corneal thickness.

The objective of a keratectomy is to remove the portion of cornea invaded by the pterygium as far as the transparent corneal layers. The thickness of the graft must be proportional to the depth of the keratectomy, without creating steps or grooves which may be the root of complications in the post-operative.

So what can be acceptable tolerance limits between the depth of the keratectomy and the thickness of the graft? The best results have been obtained when the thickness of the flap is equal to or slightly less than the depth of the keratectomy; a thicker graft will give the patient a foreign body

sensation and trophic disturbances of the tissue; on the other hand, a graft that is excessively thin will be sunken and will produce irregular astigmatism in addition to a certain degree of irregularity of the pre-corneal lacrimal film. A moderate difference in thickness is the rule in this type of surgery but it is generally well-tolerated.

BIOLOGICAL FEATURES OF THE GRAFT

Biologically and clinically, the ideal graft material for lamellar keratoplasty consists of a "fresh" corneal graft prepared directly in the operating room with the tissue removed from a globe that has just been explanted. However, in reality, discs of dehydrated corneal tissue of a variety of sizes is increasing in popularity.

The advantages of the "fresh" tissue lie in the possibility of choosing the corneal position that is most suitable for the removal and to be able to prepare flaps of shape and depth suitable for the operation.

In our experience, the results are good with both the dehydrated and the fresh tissue. However, it must be stated that with the latter tissue, there is a more rapid return to transparency and a more rapid post-operative re-epithelialization.

PREPARATION OF THE LENTICLE

• **From an intact globe.** The eyes are stored in a humidity chamber at a temperature of +4°C. These are corneas that are not suitable for penetrating keratoplasty because of the insufficient endothelium. The biological characteristics of vitality and transparency remain unchanged. The disc of corneal tissue is obtained by trephining the corneal stroma and the subsequent trephination. The discs of corneal tissue can be used in surgery immediately after the preparation of the recipient globe; alternately they can be dehydrated and stored for later use.

• **From preserved tissue.** The dehydrated discs of corneal tissue are re-hydrated for a few minutes with physiological saline solution, prior to being used in the operating room. The re-hydration restores the transparency but the thickness is generally greater than it will be at the end of the case. In some cases, due to a lack of preserved flaps or entire globes, the graft can be obtained from sclero-limbal flaps preserved for penetrating keratoplasty; in this case, special devices - artificial anterior chambers - are used. These are sealed systems that fix the sclero-corneal button on a superior aperture on the device. By means of a syringe that injects a physiological solution into the system, positive pressure is maintained. The maneuvers of trephining and dissection can now be performed. Even though in theory the artificial anterior chambers are excellent systems, in practice, trephining and dissection prove difficult because of the loss of sealing and because of the deformation of the globe. The discs of corneal tissue, following trephining, are obtained using a hand trephine of diameter between 9.0 and 12.0 mm; generally speaking, an over-sized diameter of 0.1- 0.5 mm is preferable, for reasons we will discuss shortly. As a means of preservation, dehydration is considered to be efficacious, microbiologically safe and economical, and provides the possibility of using the tissue weeks or months later without reducing its therapeutic efficacy or compromising the transparency; in our personal clinical experience, we have obtained good results with dehydrated tissue that has been stored for up to three months.

TECHNIQUE FOR PREPARING A LAMELLAR LENTICLE FROM AN INTACT GLOBE

- **Preliminary phase.** Following the decontamination procedures with a solution of 5% Iodine-povidone for 2 minutes and the successive neutralization of the Iodine in a solution of Sodium thiosulfate for one minute, the globe is immersed in a sterile salt solution until the surgeon is ready to prepare the lenticle. The globe is removed from the saline solution and placed on a sterile

gauze which binds it at the equator; this binding allows the globe to be held firmly between the fingers to create the correct pressure and facilitate the maneuvers of trephining and dissecting. The sloughed epithelium is gently removed from the corneal surface using a damp sponge *(Figure 14-3)*.

- **Technique**

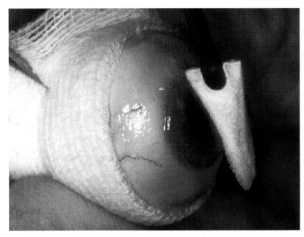

Figure 14-3. *The fresh globe is stored in a humidity chamber. It is bound with a gauze positioned at the equator which produces sufficient tension for the successive steps. A sterile sponge is used to remove the sloughed corneal epithelium.*

Practical Advice for the Preparation of the Flap

a) A regular keratectomy is used only if the corneal dissection is performed on a single plane. When the dissection proceeds smoothly the surgeon feels that he is proceeding with ease and no resistance; if he feels a certain amount of friction or a "click" during advancement, this indicates that he has changed cleavage plane.

b) Low globe pressure will encourage a deepening of the dissection; on the contrary, excess pressure will encourage a more superficial dissection.

c) In the creation of a cleavage plane, when the operator is aware that the depth is not satisfactory for the dissection of the cornea, all he has to do is create another plane in a different sector.

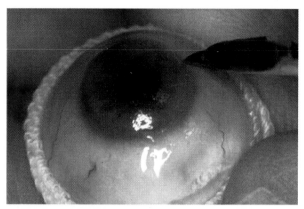

Figure 14-4. *Scalpel is used to create an incision measuring about 3-4 mm, close to the limbus for the ideal depth for the thickness we wish to obtain (between half to two-thirds of the corneal thickness). The incision must allow the insertion of the spatula that will be used for the dissection of the entire surface.*

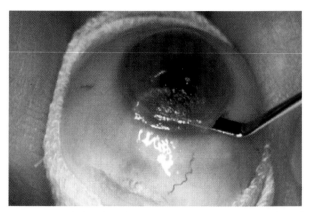

Figure 14-7. *The lamellar dissection must involve the entire surface of the cornea, reaching and exceeding the surgical limbus for the entire circle. Sometimes the length of the sharp dissection instrument is not long enough to dissect the whole cornea and peripheral dissection is completed with a blunt cyclo-dialysis spatula.*

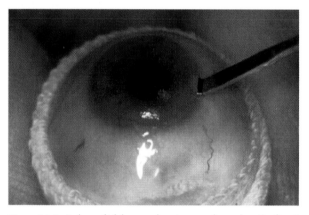

Figure 14-5. *A short, slightly curved cutting spatula, such as Paufique's spatula is introduced to the incision prepared and creates the cleavage plane of the dissection. This is a very important surgical phase because it conditions the thickness of the flap.*

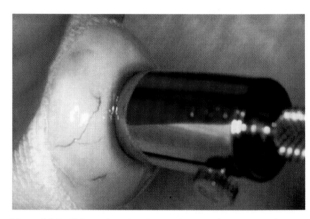

Figure 14-8. *When dissection is complete, trephination can be performed. The diameter of the trephine is chosen on the basis of the total diameter of the cornea, any senile marginal dystrophic corneal pathologies or other pathologies of the peripheral cornea. The Franceschetti hand trephine regulated for a semi-perforating cut is shown in the Figure.*

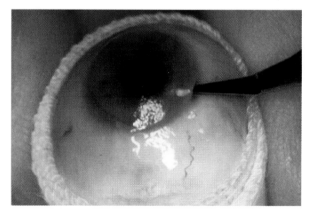

Figure 14-6. *A circular dissection spatula with cutting edges is introduced to the pouch created and completes the dissection over the entire surface of the cornea.*

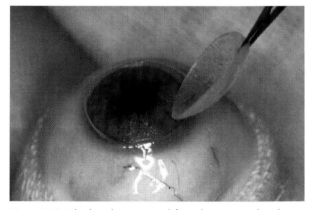

Figure 14-9. *The lenticle is removed from the cornea, placed on a support and washed with an antibiotic and physiological solution. The flap is ready for use or storage.*

d) The hand trephine should be adjusted for a semi penetrating cut (about 500 microns) and it must be positioned perpendicular to the corneal surface. The cut must be completed through rotation and not through pressure.

e) Following trephination, the thin slices of tissue that join the flap to the underlying stroma, caused by the change in the dissection plane or by incomplete trephination, must be cut with Vannas scissors placed parallel to the lenticle surface that is held taut with forceps.

f) The peripheral shapes and the smaller circular ones are obtained from larger corneal discs. The lenticle is placed with the stromal surface facing upwards, dried and distended, it is trephined to the diameter and shape required.

Surgical Technique of Lamellar Keratoplasty in Pterygium

Preparation of the Graft Site: Trephination and Keratectomy

Following removal of the pterygium from the corneal surface, as we have seen in the general part on surgery, the optical zone is marked with a 6 mm refractive surgery marker, while the corneal limit of the keratectomy is marked with a hand trephine chosen on the basis of the extension of the pterygium on the cornea and the previously marked optical zone.

In the central circular keratoplasty, it is not necessary to mark the optical zone.

• **Trephination: diameter and adjustment of the trephine.** Franceschetti's hand trephine adapts very well to the technique of lamellar keratoplasty thanks to its technical features and the internal piston which allows the precise adjustment of the cutting depth.
The diameter depends on the extension of pterygium on the cornea.

In a peripheral half-moon keratoplasty, the choice of the trephine diameter is a question of "trial-and-error". The surgeon "tries-out" trephines of increasing diameter (9-10-11-12 mm) until he finds the one that can cover all the damaged cornea without exceeding the limits of the optical zone that has been marked; by increasing the diameter of the trephine, the convexity of the cornea is reduced with an increase in the arc of the circle corresponding to the limbus; the opposite is true when the diameter is reduced. The diameter of the trephine must be smaller than the diameter of the graft or its radius of curvature to encourage positioning of the flap and the sutures.

In a peripheral keratoplasty, the over-sizing of the graft is 0.1 mm whereas this increases to 0.5 mm in the circular forms. Regulation of the trephine depth occurs by means of a micrometric screw fitted to the end of the trephine handle and is chosen depending on the degree of involment of the cornea.

Generally speaking, for pterygia, about one-third of the corneal thickness is removed and the regulation of the trephine is around 300 microns. In the Franceschetti trephine, this corresponds to a complete turn of the screw less two lines.

In the more involved forms and in the recurrences, a deeper keratectomy may be necessary, to as much as 2/3 of the corneal depth and the trephine will be adjusted with a complete turn of the screw - corresponding to about 500 microns *(Figures 14-10, 14-11, 14-12)*.

• **Keratectomy.** After having marked the cornea by trephination, the groove is examined to ensure that its depth is compatible with the depth of the keratectomy; a shallow cut can be deepened with cutting instruments at the point where the cleavage plane will be created. The cleavage plane is created by introducing a cutting spatula to the groove that is allowed to advance gently with alternating clockwise and anti-clockwise movements.

The instruments that have proved most useful for the creation of the cleavage plane are spatulas with cutting discs and Paufique's short, angled spatula.

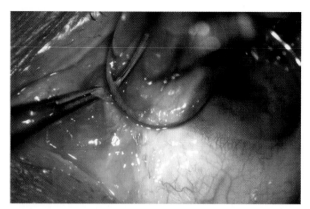

Figure 14-10. *Trephination of the lamellar keratoplasty. Peripheral trephination for a half-moon LK. The eye bulb is held in slight abduction with conjunctival forceps. Franceschetti's hand trephine, indenting the globe, produces the initial marking to show whether the diameter of the trephine is suitable for the operation.*

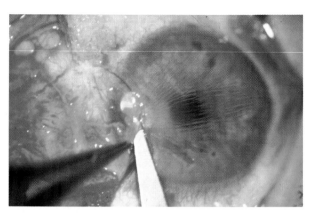

Figure 14-13. *Keratectomy. With a round cutting spatula, the surgeon completes the keratectomy from the center to the limbus and undermines the edges of the cornea to create a peripheral pouch that will be used for placing and suturing the graft.*

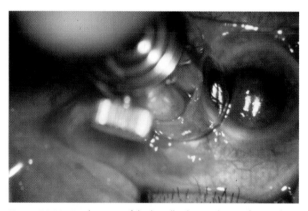

Figure 14-11. *Trephination of the lamellar keratoplasty. After marking, the surgeon checks the extension of the limbal limits and to what degree the optical zone has been saved. The trephine is returned to the groove and inclined slightly towards the cornea to accentuate the cut in this area as opposed to the sclera. Trephination has to be made rotating the handle of the trephine rather than pressing on the cornea. During trephination, the surgeon must check the position of the trephine by observing it from outside the operating field or alternately reducing the microscope magnification to a minimum.*

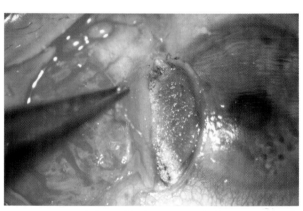

Figure 14-14. *Final phase of the keratectomy. The keratectomy is sufficiently deep and has eliminated all the opacity and any infiltration by the head of the pterygium. The surface appears porous and translucent; a small irregular area can be observed in the inferior part of the keratectomy.*

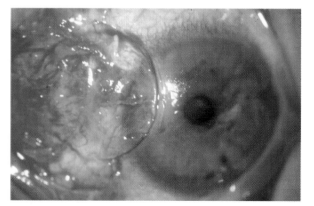

Figure 14-12. *Appearance of the cornea after trephination. A 9 mm Franceschetti's hand trephine was used in this operation. The diameter of the trephine covered the extension of the pterygium to the limbus and did not involve the optical zone.*

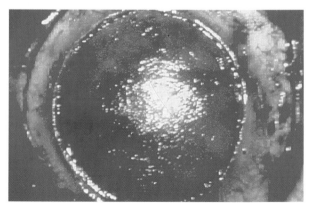

Figure 14-15. *Final phase of the keratectomy. In this operation of keratoplasty, the keratectomy was wide and deep. The surface is fairly smooth with a porous, translucent appearance.*

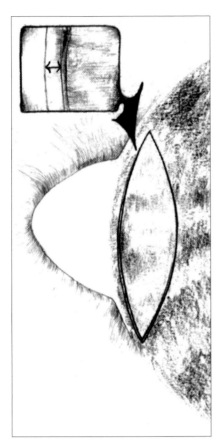

Drawing 14-8. *The drawing shows the ideal peripheral half-moon keratectomy. The details of the drawing highlight the peripheral corneal pouch necessary for the placement and suturing of the flap.*

Following dissection and removal of the involved cornea, the edges of the keratectomy are undermined full-circle to create a pouch. In the successive phases, this will facilitate bringing the graft and the suture together *(Figure 14-13).*
Following a successfully completed keratectomy, the corneal surface must be smooth, porous and translucent *(Figures 14-14, 14-15).*

Positioning and Suturing of the Graft

The graft tissue prepared previously is removed from it silicone support and placed in the keratectomy.

The positioning must be precise to allow the perfect coincidence of the edges of the graft with those of the cornea *(Figure 14-16).*

The diameter of the graft must be greater than the diameter of the keratectomy.

This over-sizing facilitates its positioning in the keratectomy and also facilitates the placement of sutures, avoiding traction, dislocation and folds. In the peripheral half-moon forms, the graft is about 0.1 mm greater whereas in the large or total keratoplasties, this difference may reach 0.5 mm.

Once the graft has been positioned, it is fixed with sutures (two at the extremities in the half-moon keratoplasties and four in the circular keratoplasties). Silk 8/0 or nylon 10/0 are used *(Figure 14-17).*

In the half-moon lamellar keratoplasty, the excess corneoscleral tissue is trimmed along the edge of the limbus using curved corneal scissors *(Figure 14-18)* and sutured in the pouch using nylon 10/0 interrupted sutures or a running stitch *(Figure 14-19).*

For the suture, very curved spatulate needles, such as the half circle, produces a smooth suture.

The needle must penetrate the flap for the full depth and enter the bottom of the peripheral pouch; this will prevent the formation of traction or torsion folds as we are sure that the tissue is sutured on the same plane.

Conjunctival plastic surgery by stretching or the simple closure of the conjunctiva terminates the operation *(Drawing 14-9).*

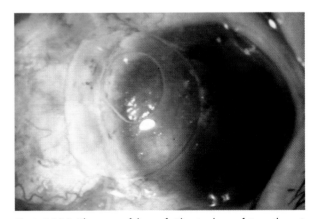

Figure 14-16. *Placement of the graft. The circular graft is easily positioned on the cornea and brought into perfect correspondence with the curved edge of the trephinated portion. In this case, the coincidence is perfect and the small air bubble at the interface improves the adaptation of the graft to the surface of the keratectomy.*

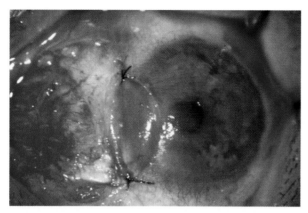

Figure 14-17. *Positioning of the graft. In this figure, the half-moon graft is placed and fixed to the limbus at the superior and inferior extremities by means of two silk 8/0 sutures. The placement of the anchoring sutures is important for the suture and prevents dislocation of the lenticle.*

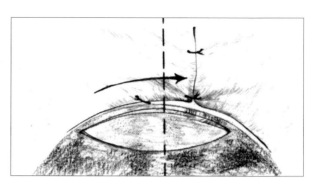

Drawing 14-9. *The drawing shows a simple technique of conjunctival repair associated with a peripheral half-moon lamellar keratoplasty. The conjunctival edges do not close on a median line at 9 o'clock on the limbus (marked by the dotted line) but slightly further down. The most proximal point to the limbus is deliberately made through the superficial layers of the sclera in order to discharge the tension and distance the conjunctiva a further 2 mm from the limbus.*

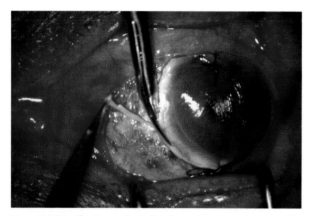

Figure 14-18. *This Figure shows the phase where, prior to suturing the graft, the surgeon trims the tissue with curved scissors along the limbal edge.*

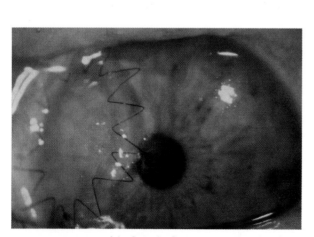

Figure 14-19. *Suture of the flap. The flap is positioned and anchored with some fixation sutures. It is then sutured with a continuous suture of 10/0 nylon. Even though the suture is regular and on the same plane, the thread must pass through the bottom of the prepared peripheral pouch.*

Practical Advice and Tips for Lamellar Keratoplasty

- **Trephination.** For precise and regular trephination, we would like to point out two important factors in relation to the inclination of the trephine and the indentation of the trephine on the globe.

In the peripheral keratoplasty, if we wish to obtain superficial trephination, the trephine must be held perpendicular to or inclined slightly on the corneal surface; on the other hand, if we wish to obtain deeper trephination, the inclination and the indentation towards the cornea must be more pronounced so that the thread of the trephine penetrates further into the cornea than it does in the sclera.

In the circular LK, the trephine must be held perpendicular and centered with precision on the cornea.

As the Franceschetti trephine lacks a system for centering, its central position must be controlled from the outside and under low magnification, or alternately observing the position from outside the operating field.

The trephination must be completed by means of smooth alternating movements (clockwise-anti-clockwise) with the hand-piece between the thumb and fore-finger.

• **Keratectomy.** Dissecting the cornea can be facilitated by pulling gently with forceps on the tissue that is being dissected; under the effects of traction the individual corneal lamellae tend to separate along the dissection plane and are clearly visible as a translucent reflection.

The keratectomy must progress along a single plane of the cornea and the surgeon feels this as a ease of advancement of the spatula; however, if there is a change in the cleavage plane, the surgeon will feel a momentary obstruction to the progression and a "click" that results from the rupture of the corneal fibers that have been ruptured as opposed to separated.

In the large peripheral or circular keratoplasties, the dissection must extend beyond the trephined edge, both in the cornea and in the sclera.

This maneuver creates a pouch around the keratectomy which has the precise purpose of facilitating the placement of the over-sized flap, optimizing the coaptation of the graft tissue and creating a suture that is on the same plane for every pass.

At the end of the keratectomy, the surgeon must observe the appearance of the corneal surface; it must be smooth, porous, translucent and free from strips of tissue.

Sunken or raised areas indicate an irregular keratectomy that has not been created on a single plane. In these cases it is necessary to smooth the surfaces to avoid complications with irritating post-operative disturbances.

The keratectomy can be smoothed in a number of ways: using a cutting spatula which trims the excess tissue, or a spatulate needle mounted on a needle holder which identifies the dissection plane with the tip while the cutting edges complete the dissection.

When the irregularity involves the central area of the cornea, the dissection can be facilitated by reducing the globe pressure by means of a small paracentesis performed with a spatulate needle that penetrates the anterior chamber on exit from a tunnel.

• **Preparation and placement of the flap.** The graft must be larger than the keratectomy. In a peripheral LK, 0.1 mm greater is sufficient while for the circular forms the increase in size can be as much as 0.5 mm.

The thickness of the lenticle should coincide with the depth of the keratectomy to avoid unacceptable discrepancies.

There are considerable difficulties in placing the graft when the shape of the flap and the keratectomy include acute angles. "Key-hole" shapes and "segments of a washer" shapes create considerable problems both with the closure and the suture. The flap can be sutured with either continuous or interrupted sutures. The needle must penetrate the full depth of the lenticle and enter the bottom of the pouch created in the cornea and/or in the sclera surrounding the keratectomy. This will greatly facilitate the phases of placement, closure and suturing of the flap. We use nylon 10/0 suture mounted on a half-circle needle (Alcon CU5).

The suture in nylon 10/0 is removed 2-3 months later.

POST-OPERATIVE COURSE AND THERAPY

Post-operative therapy consists of broad spectrum antibiotic eye-drops such as aminoglycosides (Netilmicin) for the first five days, in association with artificial tear (Sodium Hyaluronate) and NSAIDs (Indomethacin) to reduce the post-operative inflammation.

When the re-epithelialization of the lenticle is complete, topical cortisone is also associated administered three times a day. The use of cortisone is contraindicated during the first 72 hours as these drugs tend to inhibit the repair processes of the corneal epithelium.

The cortisone/antibiotic association must be continued for at least one month after surgery. If the suture material used in the conjunctiva is non-absorbable, it must be removed about 7-10 days; nylon sutures need to be removed 2-3 months from the operation.

COMPLICATIONS OF LAMELLAR KERATOPLASTY

The complications can be split into intra-operative and post-operative.

Intraoperative Complications

- **Corneal perforation.** This complication may occur during the trephination or keratectomy phases. It is an unlikely occurrence with trephination if the trephine is fitted with a central block but is a possibility if the cut depth has not been set correctly. In this case it is necessary to suture the edges of the perforation with nylon 10/0 and postpone the operation to a later date. Perforation is more likely to occur during keratectomy, particularly in the phases of repeated deepening and smoothing of the surface. If the perforation causes the infiltration of aqueous humor into the corneal stroma, the tissue must be returned to its original site, sutured and the operation suspended. The introduction of an air bubble to the anterior chamber will reduce the infiltration of aqueous humor to the interface, prevents the reduction of the anterior chamber and facilitates the closure of the perforation. A micro-perforation that closes spontaneously, rapidly and without filtration of the aqueous humor consents non-urgent treatment and it very often happens that the operation can be terminated as planned. Special attention should be paid in the keratectomy performed on pterygia treated previously with Mitomycin C or following Strontium 90 therapy. In the cornea below the head of the pterygium, these two forms of treatment may cause cornea thinning or sloughed or dystrophic zones that tend to scar very slowly. In these situations, a perforation is more frequent and is a very serious situation to manage because the mechanisms for tissue repair are inhibited or have been slowed down. In these cases, in addition to replacing and suturing the tissue that is being carved, the surgeon should cover the perforated area by stretching the conjunctiva. He should avoid using the nasal conjunctiva, where the body of the pterygium is normally found, and which is almost cer-

tainly involved in the negative effects of the antimitotic treatment. On some rare occasions, when the keratectomy or the suture are being placed, the needle penetrates the anterior chamber causing an infiltration of aqueous humor to the interface which may go unnoticed. Under these circumstances, the filtration may form a bag or pseudo-chamber that may expand in the post-operative and prevent adhesion between the corneal surfaces; sometimes, it may become infected with serious consequences to the globe. The treatment of these complications involves introducing a large air bubble to the anterior chamber which acts as a tamponade on the infiltration and pushes the cornea towards the flap. These mechanisms generally provide a rapid solution to the case.

- **Step between the graft and the surrounding cornea.** When the graft tissue is considerably thinner than the depth of the keratectomy, the entire zone will be sunken. This will reduce the therapeutic barrier effect created by the lamellar keratoplasty but above all induces irregular astigmatism that may be severe and which provokes the irritating phenomena of diffraction.

The phenomena of diffraction are accentuated by the uneven distribution of the lacrimal film over the sunken area.

The astigmatism induced by surgery can be observed and evaluated simply by using corneal topography.

With thick flaps, this can be avoided by deepening the keratectomy layer by layer until a depth compatible with the thickness of the graft is achieved. It is difficult to obtain the perfect coincidence between the depth of the keratectomy and the thickness of the graft but minor level differences are acceptable and compatible.

A thicker flap produces a constant foreign body sensation caused by the tactile sensation perceived by the eyelid on the raised corneal zone; this symptom generally diminishes and disappears within three months from surgery. Finally it should also be pointed out that the shape of the graft does not always coincide perfectly with the shape of the keratectomy and may produce an irregular junction line. Following scar forma-

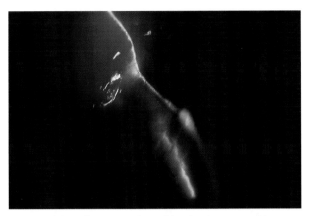

Figure 14-20. In this patient, the problem has been caused by excessively thin graft tissue. The fissure clearly shows the subsidence of the graft and the formation of a concavity that produces a dellen effect due to an alteration of the lacrimal film.

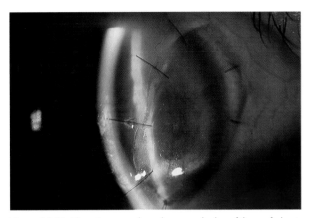

Figure 14-23. There is a step along the corneal edge of the graft due to the peripheral pouch that is excessively small.

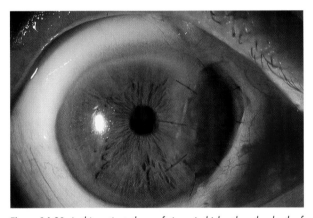

Figure 14-21. In this patient, the graft tissue is thicker than the depth of the keratectomy. Attachment and transparency are normal but the patient complains of a constant, uncomfortable foreign body sensation caused by the raised edge of the graft tissue from the corneal surface. There is also a certain degree of irregularity in the corneal profile of the flap caused by an excess in the central profile, not compensated by the shallow peripheral pouch.

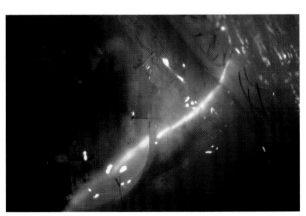

Figure 14-22. Irregularity of the graft. The thickness of the flap is excessive because of an excessively superficial keratectomy. The treatment of this complication involves the removal of the graft, further deepening of the keratectomy and the peripheral pouch.

tion, this may induce irregular astigmatism that is difficult to treat *(Figures 14-20, 14-21, 14-22, 14-23).*

• **Perforation of the flap.** This is the result of careless manipulation of the flap during placement on the cornea. A micro-perforation will not affect the final outcome of the operation but a macro-perforation is not acceptable and the flap must be replaced.

• **Hemorrhage**. Cutting the vessels in the head or in the body of pterygium always causes bleeding that makes the completion of the keratectomy difficult. In these cases, the surgeon can perform episcleral coagulation as far as the limbus or alternately, he can apply to the bleeding a fragment of sponge soaked in a 1:100,000 solution of adrenaline or a 10% solution of phenylephrine.

• **Upside-down placement of the graft.** This is a very rare occurrence which can also pass unnoticed. In some cases, it may be suspected for the porous effect of the graft surface, because of the delayed epithelialization associated with a very smooth, even interface, or because of epithelialization of the interface.

• **Irregular suture.** A continuous, superficial or relaxed suture will cause sometime intolerable irritation that sometimes necessitates the early removal of the sutures, even just a few weeks after surgery.

In those cases where the keratectomy has not created a peripheral pouch, the suture can cause traction folds or everted or sunken areas. These folds are almost always formed when the suture passes (continuous or interrupted) are not on the same plane. In these cases, if the closure creates differences in level of the graft, there may be aberrations from scarring which require the removal of the suture. The flap must be peeled back partially or totally, a peripheral pouch must be created or the existing one deepened, and the flap re-sutured.

- **Foreign body at the interface.** This is a frequent occurrence and normally consists of fragments of inert material from the sterile drapes, fine powder or small fragments of suture thread.

  If a fragment of silk or other reactive material is trapped at the interface, it should be removed by washing the interface with a solution delivered by a fine cannula. The interface should be washed and checked at the end of each operation as part of routine practice.

Post-operative Complications

- **Separation of the wound**

  There are a number of reasons:

  1. defect in the suture
  2. post-operative contusion
  3. massive hemorrhage at the interface
  4. premature removal of the suture
  5. scar defects
  6. infection of the edges.

  Treatment must be decided on the basis of the cause. A small dehiscence will close spontaneously and will not create problems whereas a suture that is completely and prematurely relaxed and causes considerable dehiscence must be removed and repeated.

- **Dislocation of the graft**. This is a rare situation which may be observed in the week immediately after surgery. The dislocation is normally nasal and leaves a portion of the corneal stroma uncovered. This complication is normally caused by the relaxation and the early precocious rupture of the suture due to trauma. If the flap is transparent, it simply needs to be re-positioned and re-sutured. However, if it is edematous, it would be better to replace it *(Figures 14-24, 14-25)*.

- **Infection**. This complication was very common in the past. Tarr reports four cases of endophthalmitis from Pseudomonas aeruginosa in a series of 63 cases of LK for pterygium, and other cases have been reported in the literature following LK for pterygium and treatment with Mitomycin C. Relaxed sutures or interrupted sutures may be the starting point of many infections *(Figures 14-26, 14-27)*.

- **Epithelialization of the interface**. This is normally secondary to a large dehiscence or the partial dislocation of the flap, or more unusually because the flap has been overturned. The treatment consists of removing the flap, scraping and washing the bed and the posterior face of the flap.

- **Fistula of the interface**. This may be caused by:

  1. Perforation of the bed during the keratectomy
  2. Filtration along the perforating pass of the suture
  3. Flaps that are much larger than the keratectomy. It is treated by placing a compression patch on the eye and introducing an air bubble to the anterior chamber if required.

- **Hemorrhage at the interface**. This is a frequent occurrence and will usually regress spontaneously within a couple of days. Sometimes the blood pool will create a persistent hemorrhage bag at the interface which may detach the flap. In these cases, the interface must aspirated and washed with an irrigation cannula *(Figure 14-28)*.

- **Deposits at the interface**. In those cases where the keratectomy does not remove the newly formed blood vessels at the head of pterygium or if these vessels re-appear at the interface during the post-operative period, some time later a lipid and cholesterol exudate may be observed that will tend to crystallize at the interface *(Figures 14-29, 14-30)*.

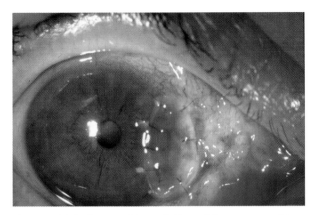

Figure 14-24. *Dislocation of the graft. The graft has an excess of tissue at the limbus which caused relaxation of a suture. This resulted in raising of the surrounding area and nasal dislocation of the lenticle.*

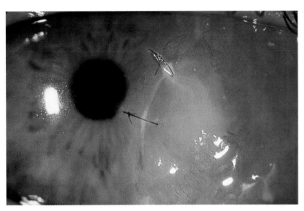

Figure 14-27. *Infection. Three weeks from surgery, this patient developed a bacterial infection with a purulent pool at the interface. The infection developed because one of the sutures relaxed.*

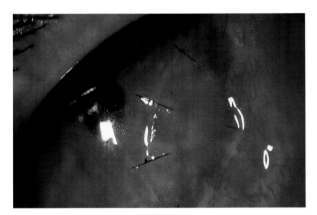

Figure 14-25. *Raising of the graft. This patient was operated on ten days previously and some of the central interrupted sutures have relaxed, causing the graft to rise, which caused considerable irritation. Treatment consists of removal of the sutures, re-positioning of the edges of the graft and replacement sutures.*

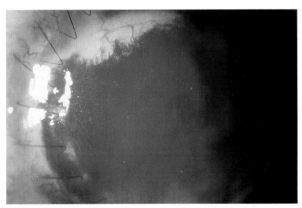

Figure 14-28. *Hemorrhage at the interface. Major hemorrhage, which appeared in the week following surgery. It involves 90% of the interface. The bright red color indicates that we are dealing with a fine layer which does not create tension in the sutures or cause dislocation of the flap. Absorption is spontaneous and no additional medical therapy is required.*

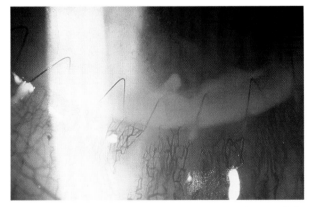

Figure 14-26. *Infection. The picture shows an infection from Staphylococcus aureus which appeared 40 days after wide lamellar keratoplasty surgery. There are signs of strong ocular congestion and septic infiltration of the suture tract. In these cases the sutures must be removed immediately and the patient subjected to antibiotic treatment specific for the bacteria.*

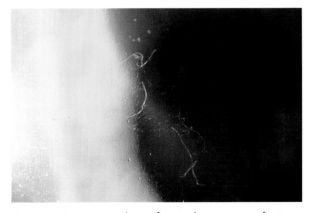

Figure 14-29. *Deposits at the interface. Under strong magnification at the slit lamp, some foreign bodies can be seen at the interface. This is a frequent occurrence in this type of surgery and usually does not cause problems of intolerance.*

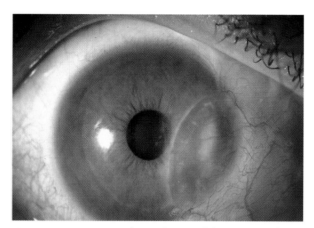

Figure 14-30. *Deposits at the interface. Lipid deposits, secondary to neo-vascularization at the interface.*

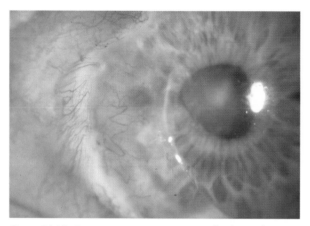

Figure 14-31. *Post-operative astigmatism. Lamellar keratoplasty nine months after surgery. Despite this shape being chosen to increase the diameter of the optical zone, there is 2.5 D of irregular astigmatism. There is also vascularization of the interface.*

- **Post-operative astigmatism.** In peripheral lamellar keratoplasty the optical zone must not be involved in the trephination and keratectomy maneuvers. The marking of an optical zone measuring 5.5 - 6.0 mm is a preliminary step of the peripheral keratoplasty. This diameter must always be respected so that uncomfortable astigmatism is avoided. A large circular lamellar keratoplasty generally does not create severe astigmatism and can normally be treated in the post-operative by the re-distribution of the suture tension. In the half-moon LK, when the edge of the graft invades the optical zone, irregular astigmatism may be created that is difficult to treat. In these cases, subsequent treatment of the optical zone with a central manual or mechanized LK, or alternately a photoablative treatment with the excimer laser may improve vision. A contact lens is not well-tolerated *(Figures 14-31, 14-32).*

- **Pterygoid scar.** This is the invasion of conjunctival fibrovascular tissue on the cornea to the limits of trephination.
  The lesion originates from where the pterygium was removed but in this case it is a newly-formed conjunctival repair tissue and is not evolutive. This rare complication is very similar to a recurrent pterygium and the differential diagnosis may prove extremely difficult *(Figure 14-33).*

- **Corneal rejection.** The homologous corneal flap contains "foreign" antigens that may cause rejec-

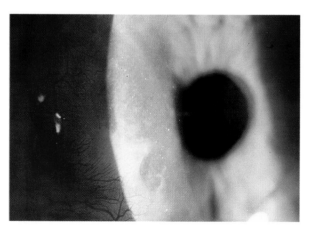

Figure 14-32. *Post-operative astigmatism. In this case, the corneal edge of a half-moon graft has involved the optical zone creating highly irregular corneal astigmatism which is difficult to treat.*

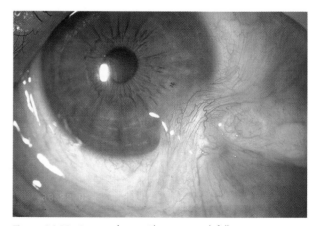

Figure 14-33. *Pterygoid scar. This appeared following a pyogenic granuloma following removal of pterygium Type I. The differential diagnosis with the recurrence is difficult but this is not an evolving complication.*

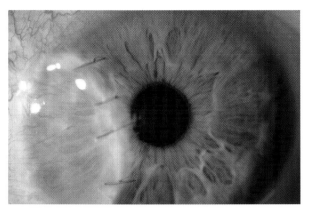

Figure 14-34. *Suspected rejection. Edema in the flap and vasculariza-tion of the interface appeared 40 days after surgery. An edematous flap following a period of transparency, accompanied by vasculariza-tion of the surface or of the interface may suggest rejection of the graft tissue. This patient was subjected to cortisone treatment and the return to transparency served to confirm the suspicion.*

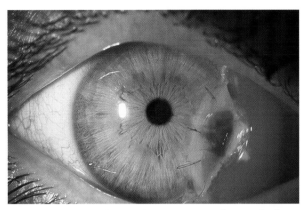

Figure 14-36. *Flap melting. In this very rare complication, the flap is subjected to a progressive destruction of the tissue with total failure of the keratoplasty. In this patient, a few days after surgery, progressive and widespread edema appeared in the flap for no apparent reason. The rapid onset and the absence of response to cortisone treatment allows immune mechanisms to be excluded.*

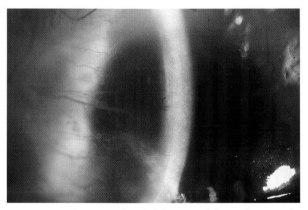

Figure 14-35. *The picture of epithelial rejection following large circular lamellar keratoplasty in recurrent pterygium Type III. Four months from surgery, an immune reaction appeared characterized by peripheral neo-vascularization of the graft with widespread edema. The inflamma-tory reaction responded well to topical steroid treatment, confirming the diagnosis.*

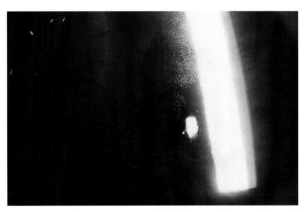

Figure 14-37. *The same patient at the slit lamp and magnified. Small inflammatory deposits can be observed in the endothelium.*

tion. In our experience, this complication is very rare (about 1% of cases); however, Rougier re-ported an incidence of around 4%.

The fact that it is such a rare occurrence may be explained by the following:

– the low number of cells (though the number is greater in fresh tissue)
– the graft tissue is thin (lower antigenicity)
– the lack of blood vessels.

Opacity of the flap with edema which appears after a period of transparency may indicate rejec-tion. It is associated with the appearance of newly-formed limbal and peripheral vessels in the graft which simulates the recurrence of ptery-gium.

Rapid response to topical steroid therapy is an important differentiation factor *(Figures 14-34, 14-35).*

• **Vascularization.** This is the growth of capillaries that surround the graft without crossing it.

This phenomenon represents an indirect clinical sign of the barrier effect produced by the periph-eral lamellar keratoplasty. The vascularization may involve the interface, but this is not a serious complication and rarely evolutive; it may result in lipid desposits at the interface *(Figure 14-30).*

- **Flap melting**. This is a very rare early post-operative complication and must be treated by replacing the flap. Bacterial infections or toxins with considerable cell-lysis properties (proteinases or collagenases) are usually to blame; however iatrogenic toxicity from the drugs or preservatives used cannot be totally excluded *(Figures 14-36, 14-37).*

VARIATIONS OF LAMELLAR KERATOPLASTY IN PTERYGIUM

The variants in pterygium involve the peripheral lamellar keratoplasty:

Troutman's Technique (1974)

- **Anesthesia**. The author recommends retrobulbar anesthesia with akinesia of the orbicular or alternately, general anesthesia can be used.

- **Surgical steps.** After the globe has been abducted, a silk 6/0 suture is passed under the belly of the pterygium.
  A spatula is used to remove the corneal epithelium for about 2 mm around the head to clearly expose the area of corneal involvement around the head of the pterygium.
  Scissors are used to create two conjunctival incisions, superior and inferior, starting from the limbus and proceeding along the edges of the body of the pterygium to reach the medial canthus.
  The scissors are then introduced under the two incisions and the body is detached from the underlying episcleral surface.
  Following detachment, Troutman curved scissors with the concavity towards the cornea are used to create a vertical cut that follows the curvature of the cornea. This is created about 2 mm from the limbus, between the two radial cuts.

- **Corneal Step.** Using conjunctival forceps, the remaining part of the body close to the limbus is raised and with a dissection spatula, for example a disc knife or bevel-up, the surgeon proceeds to

cut towards the cornea just beyond the apex of the pterygium.
This dissection must be superficial in poorly-evolved pterygia where a lamellar corneal graft has not been scheduled; in evolved pterygia, the corneal area to be removed with the Franceschetti trephines is outlined and the keratectomy is completed plane-by-plane.
The author suggests preparation of the flap with the same trephine used to outline the keratectomy and to use a running suture in nylon 10/0 after the placement of silk 5/0 interrupted anchor sutures.

- **Repair of the conjunctiva**. The remainder of the body of the pterygium is detached from the fibrovascular tissue and sutured with nylon 10/0 or Vicryl 8/0 to the surrounding conjunctiva, distancing it about 3 mm from the limbus.
  In the event that mobilization of the conjunctival flap proves difficult, the author recommends a free graft of autologous conjunctiva. Alternately, the surgeon can leave the exposed scleral surface to spontaneous scarring.[97]

Heilman-Paton Technique (1987)

- **Anesthesia.** Retrobulbar with akinesia or general anesthesia

- **Preparation.** The operation begins with the excision of the head and the entire body of the pterygium in one piece.

- **Corneal step.** The keratectomy is performed on a peripheral half-moon portion of the cornea to include the entire head, the front of the pterygium and the tissue immediately surrounding it. The limit of the keratectomy is not outlined by any instrument but is performed by means of a free-hand pre-incision using a blade and continued as far as the limbus with a cutting spatula.
  The cut to the limbus must be performed with curved scissors to follow the limbal curve.
  The flap for grafting is prepared from discs of tissue of diameter 10 mm. A vertical cut is performed to create a segment of a circle. The flap is placed on the corneal bed and sutured with interrupted sutures in nylon 10/0 with embedded

knots. If the corneal edge is uneven, or if there is excess tissue limbal edge, these must be trimmed with curved corneal scissors.

- **Repair of the conjunctiva.** This is performed with a stretch conjunctival plastic, which creates a square flap from the inferior bulbar conjunctiva which is pulled upwards. The suture to the surrounding conjunctiva must leave a portion of the sclera in front of the limbus exposed.

This area should prevent excessive conjunctival scarring and minimize the interruption to the lacrimal film and the formation of a dellen.

Townsend's Technique (1988)

- **Anesthesia.** Retrobulbar or peribulbar

- **Corneal step.** When the pterygium is small, a peripheral half-moon keratectomy is performed. If it is larger and invades the optical zone to a greater degree, the author recommends a trapezoidal keratectomy.

A free-hand corneal pre-incision is performed with a disposable blade, or using a pre-calibrated or adjustable knife. The incision must be linear and vertical so that it outlines a segment of a circle that is convex at the limbus.

When the pterygium is extremely large, the vertical central incision must be shorter and continued to the limbus by means of two longer radial incisions. From the author's experience, this shape of incision reduces damage to the optical zone because this area is less involved by the suture line and the resulting scar line. The author suggests checking that the edges of the keratectomy are steep so that the flap can be placed in proximity and sutured well to the surrounding cornea.

The corneal flap is prepared from dehydrated tissue discs measuring 9-10 or 12 mm of thickness 0.3 mm.

The discs of tissue are rehydrated with a saline and antibiotic solution (Gentamycin 100 mg/ml) for 20 minutes.

The diameter is chosen by placing a button of 9-10 mm on the surface of the keratectomy bringing it close to the internal edge of this; if the circumference of the flap matches that of the keratectomy for 3-4 clock hours, the diameter is correct; however, if the flap matches for more than 4 clock hours, larger flaps should be used (12 mm).

The flap is sutured with some interrupted sutures and if the position is considered to be correct, the surgeon proceeds with interrupted suture points of 10/0 nylon. The excess tissue beyond the limbus is removed with curved scissors to produce the definitive shape of the graft.[4]

LAMELLAR KERATOPLASTY WITH THE MICROKERATOME

The lamellar keratoplasty (LK) involves the replacement of a layer of opaque, altered, superficial cornea with an equivalent layer of transparent cornea from a donor globe. The operation can be performed with manual dissection or with the microkeratome. The manual operation is not used frequently as it results in uneven, non-homogeneous surfaces and inaccurate flap thickness.

In 1991, C. Genisi was the first surgeon to perform the lamellar keratoplasty with a microkeratome as a routine technique in keratoconus (Lamellar keratoplasty with differentiated thickness).

Then L. Buratto performed a similar procedure using the excimer laser (ELLKAT - Excimer Laser Lamellar Keratoplasty of Augmented Thickness).

Preparation of the Homoplastic Disc from Donor Tissue

A microkeratome is used to prepare a disc of superficial cornea from an intact donor globe or from a cornea mounted on an artificial anterior chamber.

If the globe is intact, the surgeon places it in a "Globe Holder" which will hold the globe firmly and increase the internal pressure. The microkeratome is then used to perform the lamellar cut of suitable thickness and diameter.

On the other hand, if the surgeon has only the cornea with the surrounding scleral ring, he places the tissue on an artificial anterior chamber. This instrument allows simulation of the conditions of the globe. Pressure can be applied to the cornea to increase the tension, resulting in an excellent quality of the lamellar cut with the microkeratome.

Normally the surgeon aims for a lamella of thickness 180 microns for a diameter of 8.5 - 10.0, in proportion to the diameter of the lamella that he expects to remove from the patient affected by pterygium.

If the globe or the cornea is fresh and the patient has already been prepared for surgery, the operation can be performed immediately. The use of fresh tissue carries with it the advantage for the patient of more rapid anatomical and functional healing.

If the operation has been planned at a later date, the disc can be stored in a number of ways.

If the operation has been planned within the space of a few hours, the flap can be stored in a humid atmosphere, in the refrigerator. In this case, the cell vitality is maintained and the post-operative healing time will be fast.

If the operation has been planned at a later stage, the disc of homoplastic tissue can be stored under silica gel which will dehydrate the tissue. In this case, the cell vitality is completely destroyed and the process of anatomical and functional healing will be prolonged. The advantage is that the flap can be preserved for at least 4-6 weeks.

A third alternative is to prepare a flap of tissue at the cryolathe and then lyophilize the tissue (Kaufman, Mc Donald technique for epikeratophakia); in this case the tissue can be preserved for several weeks before use.

Technique on the Patient

The pterygium is removed with the planned technique.

The body of the pterygium is dissected from the scleral surface and the conjunctival and sub-conjunctival scar tissue carefully removed.

The pterygium and the nasal conjunctiva must be removed in such a way that the suction ring of the microkeratome can adhere firmly to the globe so that the lamellar cut is perfect in terms of diameter, thickness and surface.

Special attention must be paid when smoothing the corneal stromal surface exposed by the removal of the pterygium and to the attempts to thin the cornea as little as possible in the area involved by the pterygium. Apart from anything else this will assist the microkeratome in producing lamellar corneal cut of equal thickness over the entire area involved and consequently the application of a homoplastic flap that on healing will result in a cornea of even, constant thickness.

It is best that the cut with the microkeratome starts in a temporal position to terminate in the nasal sector. It must produce a free-cap, that is, it will not have a hinge.

The suction ring of the Hansatome microkeratome is applied in a moderately decentered position so that the last part of the cut is performed in the area where the pterygium has caused greater alteration of the cornea.

The diameter of the ring - 8.5, 9.5 or 10.0 ring is chosen either in proportion to the diameter of the cornea but more specifically in relation to the extension of the pterygium. Prior to proceeding with the lamellar cut, the surgeon must ensure that the ring has adhered firmly to the globe. He must also make sure that the ocular pressure has been increased sufficiently.

The microkeratome then performs the lamellar keratotomy with a 180 micron head. The cut must be performed without a hinge being created; if the ACS is used, the cut is performed using the normal technique with the cut decentered nasally.

Placement of the Disc

The disc of homoplastic tissue is removed from its container (a tub of silica gel or a bottles containing the lyophilized flap) and washed abundantly. It is dehydrated for five minutes in a saline solution containing gentamycin (100 mcg/ml) to restore the normal degree of hydration, thickness and transparency.

It is applied to the patient's cornea that has already been subjected to a lamellar cut with the microkeratome. The surgeon must ensure that the cut diameter coincides with that of the homoplastic flap. In the event of discrepancies, the tissue must be adjusted, undermining the receiving cornea so that the donor flap slides into the circular pouch obtained.

In the nasal sector where the pterygium has been removed, it may be necessary to apply an extra fragment of corneal tissue, beside the circular tissue obtained with the microkeratome.

The flap is then sutured.

Suture

The suture serves to immobilize the flap in the correct position.

The suture begins with the placement of four interrupted sutures that center and stabilize the flap on the receiving bed. Then another four sutures are placed symmetrically. Another eight sutures are required (or alternately a continuous anti-torque suture) to allow the peripheral flap to adhere well to the receiving bed and avoid that the epithelium infiltrates below the flap itself.

The sutures must be radial and of equal tension. The knot must be rotated and buried in the tissue.

Intraoperative keratoscopy is very useful for reducing post-operative astigmatism.

The interrupted sutures allow the surgeon to adjust the astigmatism in the immediate post-operative period.

Comments

The technique of lamellar keratoplasty with the microkeratome has a series of advantages over the manual technique.

The quality of the final result is strongly influenced by the quality of the cutting surfaces and the consequent quality of the interface.

Above all, the microkeratome allows resections with smooth, even surfaces.

Moreover, the calculation of the thicknesses and the diameter of the lamellae (both donor tissue and on the patient's eye) is more precise and predictable; moreover, the operation is completed more rapidly.

In conclusion, this technique today is the valid alternative to the normal techniques of lamellar keratoplasty for the treatment of recurrent pterygium, because the normal technological developments of the latest generations of microkeratomes have brought about an important contribution to improving the quality of the cut surfaces.

15

Surgery of Pterygium With Limbal Grafts

Introduction

Limbal surgery of a pterygium that involves the use of free grafts of conjunctival tissue is considered to be one of the barrier techniques, that is the techniques that attempt to block the recurrences. The main indications for this technique are evolving recurrent pterygia, both Type II and Type III, which are the clinical forms with the highest percentage of recurrences.

The free conjunctival tissue graft to the limbus terminates the operation for pyterigium removal, or alternately peripheral or central lamellar keratoplasty.

The validity of limbal grafts has been unanimously accepted and studies on the physiopathology of the limbus confirm the theory that this anatomical transition zone, in addition to having important functions in the reproduction and regulation of the corneal epithelium turnover, creates a valid barrier to pathogenetic stimuli and the expansion of pathologies from the conjunctiva.

A form of indirect proof is the clinical observation that in pterygium surgery, the treatment of the conjunctiva frequently leads to recurrences whereas a limbal treatment, that restores a certain degree of barrier, provides superior therapeutic results.

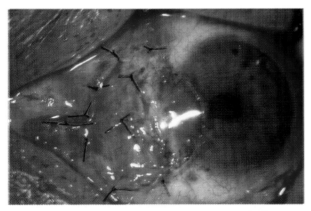

Figure 15-1. *Free graft of bulbar conjunctiva following a half-moon LK for a repeatedly recurrent pterygium Type II. The association of two techniques permits not only the potential for barrier effect but also produces favorable results in the reconstruction of the conjunctival layer and in the aesthetic result.*

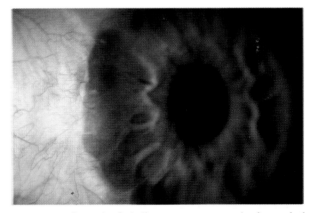

Figure 15-2. *The results of a half-moon LK operation with a free graft of limbal conjunctiva. The therapeutic and aesthetic results are excellent.*

FREE GRAFT OF CONJUNCTIVAL TISSUE

In pterygium surgery, autologous free grafts of bulbar or limbal conjunctiva are used. No studies to date have examined whether the graft of limbal conjunctiva is better than the bulbar conjunctiva. The indications are the same for both. From a physiopathological point of view, limbal conjunctiva should be better than the bulb conjunctiva because the limbal tissue is grafted to a more physiological site.

The flap of bulbar conjunctiva is removed from the superior sector of the globe; the limbal flap is removed from the superior limbus.

Various techniques of conjunctival tissue grafting have been used with pterygia in the past:

- Valierè-Vialeix technique with the autologous bulbar conjunctiva removed from the superior conjunctival fornix;

- Majoros technique where the conjunctiva is removed from the superior quadrant.

The authors justify the decision to remove the tissue from the superior sector because this sector is free from conjunctival pathologies and the pterygium itself.

At that time, the decision to use autologous conjunctival tissue was not based of knowledge of the physiology of the limbus but was simply considered to be a means of replacing the missing conjunctiva following considerable excision of the body of the pterygium.

In the original techniques, a flap measuring 5 x 5 mm was placed on the sclera behind the limbus and positioned without the need for sutures where the pterygium had been excised. It was left to dry for about 15 minutes to prevent wrinkling or dislocation. In the techniques used today, the graft is not allowed to dry to avoid damaging the conjunctival cells or creating necrosis in the graft tissue which would eliminate any therapeutic benefit of the operation.

• Removal and Graft

Following the removal of pterygium and the coagulation of the scleral vessels, the surface that remains exposed is measured using a compass or a millimetric ruler. The patient is asked to look downwards (if topical anesthesia has been used) or the globe is pushed down to expose the conjunctiva from the limbus to the fornix.

The limits of tissue removal can be marked using a dermographic pen. In order to facilitate the tissue removal, the layer of conjunctiva can be separated from the episcleral layer by infiltration of an anesthetic or physiological solution, taking care not to infiltrate the episcleral space which would make the surgical maneuvers more difficult due to the excessive mobility of the tissue.

Conjunctival forceps raise the surface conjunctiva which is cut with pointed scissors to create a small opening that is wide enough for the introduction of the scissor arms. The conjunctiva is peeled back from the episclera and the conjunctival flap is cut.

The cut flap is carefully placed on the cornea with the epithelial surface facing upwards; it is then positioned in the graft site. It is of the utmost importance that the maneuvers of tissue removal and handling of the flap are performed carefully and gently to avoid tearing, cutting or damaging the thin mucosa.

If the sampling site bleeds, it must be coagulated and allowed to re-epitelialize spontaneously, alternately the edges can be sutured with an absorbable material.

The technique used to remove of the limbal flap does not differ considerably from the technique used for the bulbar conjunctiva.

For the removal of limbal tissue, some authors[105] suggest dissecting a thin layer of peripheral cornea with the conjunctiva.

Following removal, the flap is positioned on the sclera and fixed to the over- and underlying limbal conjunctiva with two interrupted sutures; the suture must be placed in accordance with the rules for a plastic surgery repair to avoid traction and allow continuity in both the graft and the surrounding conjunctiva *(Figure 15-1)*. Vicryl 7/0 rapid, silk 8/0 or nylon 9/0-10/0 are the most suitable suture materials.

Post-operative therapy consists of topical antibiotic eyedrops three times a day for the initial 72 hours (fluorquinolones or chloramphenicol are preferred because of the lower degree of epithelial toxicity). An artificial tear (sodium hyaluronate or derivatives of methylcellulose) is applied every three hours.

Cortisone treatment, three times a day, is started from Day 4 and continued for 2-3 weeks. The non-absorbable suture is removed after 7-10 days (silk 8/0) or 10-14 days (nylon 9/0-10/0).

The post-operative course is usually uneventful. During the first few days post-operatively, the graft will appear pale as there are few blood vessels but over the following weeks it will assume the pinkish color of normal conjunctiva.

Re-vascularization is rapid and starts 24 hours from the graft operation.

The complications are comparable to those of a plastic surgery repair.

If the flap is positioned upside down, the benefits of the graft will be eliminated through the loss of trophism of the graft.

Grafting a Flap of Conjunctival Tissue Associated With the Amniotic Membrane

It would appear to be very interesting and will be covered later in the book.

Surgery of primary or recurrent pterygium with the techniques of mucosal grafting is widespread and is still wide open in research terms.

RESULTS

Surgery of a pterygium with a free graft of autologous conjunctival tissue has proved efficacious in reducing the number of recurrences observed 12 months after treatment: 2.6% in the primary forms and 9.1% in the recurrent forms (109), with aesthetically acceptable results: a few months after surgery, the thin flap of graft tissue is indistinguishable from the surrounding conjunctiva *(Figure 15-3)*.

A number of similar techniques have been described that differ through some minor variations or modifications.

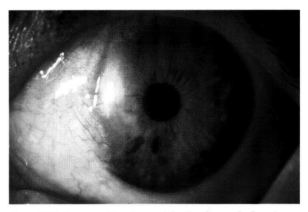

Figure 15-3. *Pterygium Type II operated with a free graft of autologous bulbar conjunctiva. The clinical picture three months after surgery. The therapeutic effect is obvious with an excellent barrier effect at the limbus. However, the problem of the corneal opacity persists and can be treated easily at a later stage.*

16

PLASTIC SURGERY TO REPAIR THE CONJUNCTIVA

INTRODUCTION

It is necessary to repair the conjunctiva following the removal of a pterygium. This applies to all techniques except scleral baring where the main feature is the spontaneous scar formation of the scleral surface.

When deciding on the most suitable technique for the specific case, the surgeon must consider the extension of the surface to be repaired, the quantity of sub-conjunctival fibrous tissue and the mucous material available for the purpose.

Of all the techniques described, we will ignore those that we feel do not satisfy the needs for efficacy and simplicity, or that in our experience have not provided good aesthetic results.

In this section, we will report only on the easier techniques which can be used in all surgical conditions and which offer acceptable aesthetic results.

CZERMAK'S TECHNIQUE

This technique repairs the conjunctiva; it brings the edges of the conjunctiva closer together and reduces traction on the flaps.

Once the conjunctiva around the damaged sclera has been peeled back and the two flaps have been mobilized, two incisions with curved scissors are performed from the attachment point of the conjunctiva to the limbus.

These continue upwards and downwards just

enough to allow easier approach of the edges without tension forces being created.

This technique is easy to perform and the aesthetic results are extremely good. It is suitable for repairing the triangular-shaped conjunctival defects that are not excessively large (*Drawings 16-1, 16-2, 16-3, 16-4*).

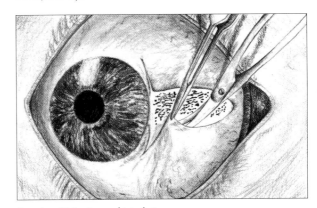

Drawing 16-1. *Czermak's technique.*

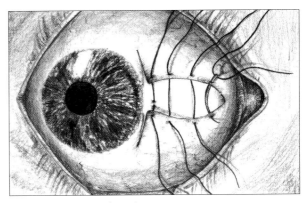

Drawing 16-2. *Czermak's technique.*

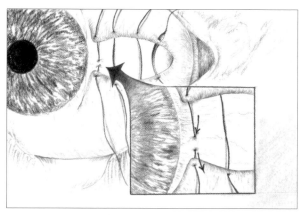

Drawing 16-3. *Czermak's technique.*

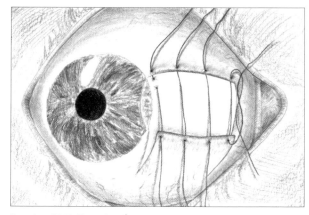

Drawing 16-5. *Terson's technique.*

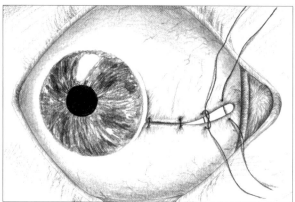

Drawing 16-4. *Czermak's technique.*

Terson's Technique

This technique is ideal for covering small surfaces, preferably rectangular or square. Following removal of the body of pterygium, two incisions several millimeters long are created along the inferior conjunctival margin and directed downwards. These incisions create a four-sided or rectangular conjunctival flap.

Once it has been detached from the underlying adhesions, it is moved upwards and sutured to the superior conjunctival edge.

The aesthetic results are excellent because the wound line is positioned above the median line and covered by the edge of the upper eyelid *(Drawing 16-5).*

Arruga's Technique

This is another technique used in the repair of small triangular conjunctival surfaces.

The flap is obtained from the superior bulbar conjunctiva by means of an incision that initially runs along the superior limbus, then it proceeds posteriorly and radially towards the conjunctival fornix.

The flap produced in this way is detached from the underlying episclera, mobilized and twisted downwards to be sutured in the repair zone.

This is an excellent technique of conjunctival plastic surgery by torsion.

It can repair larger surfaces than the Terson technique, providing good aesthetic results *(Drawings 16-6, 16-7).*

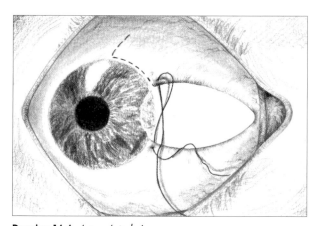

Drawing 16-6. *Arruga's technique.*

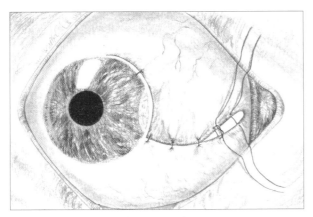

Drawing 16-7. *Final step of Arruga's technique.*

ARLT'S TECHNIQUE

Like the previous technique, a conjunctival flap is created in the superior bulbar conjunctiva. It is mobilized and allowed to run downwards in the nasal sector.

Compared to the Arruga technique, it is more suitable for rhomboid-shaped conjunctival defects, such as excision of a pterygium with a large collarette and a hypertrophic body that extends as far as the semilunar fold.

Two incisions are made along the superior edge of the conjunctiva, the first one upwards along the limbus and the other posterior towards the superior fornix.

This flap is peeled back, mobilized and moved downwards to be sutured to the lower edge of the conjunctiva *(Drawing 16-8).*

VALIERÈ-VIALEIX'S TECHNIQUE

The conjunctival flap is obtained from the bulbar conjunctiva in the supero-internal quadrant, close to the fornix. This flap is mobilized and placed on the site of the pterygium body and then sutured to the surrounding conjunctiva. The advantages of this technique are largely aesthetic with rapid and safe attachment.

STRAMPELLI'S TECHNIQUE

This does not differ greatly from the previous technique except that a small fragment of peripheral cornea is removed from the superior limbus and grafted to the nasal limbus where the head of the pterygium was located *(Drawings 16-9, 16-10).*

This can be considered to be a technique that anticipated the limbal surgery techniques by several years.

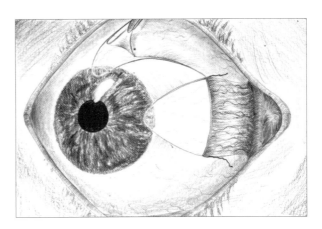

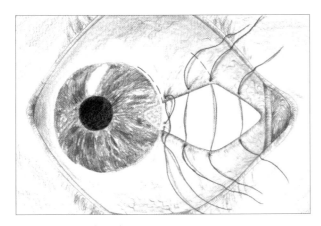

Drawing 16-8. *Arlt's technique.*

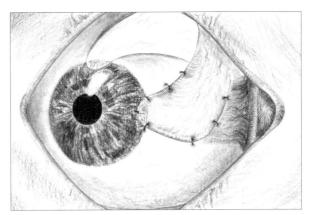

Drawings 16-9 and 16-10. *Strampelli's technique.*

GENERAL RULES FOR PLASTIC SURGERY OF THE CONJUNCTIVA

a) folds must not be created when the edges are brought together;

b) the physiological shrinkage of the conjunctival tissue must be considered when calculating the size of the surface to be repaired;

c) excessive tension in the flaps will relax the sutures and facilitate diastasis of the wound line;

d) the tissue used to cover the sclera must stop a couple of millimeters from the limbus so that a small portion of bare sclera remains uncovered;

e) in order to increase the adhesion of the conjunctiva to the underlying layers and to avoid excessive retraction with conjunctival dislocation, the conjunctiva can be anchored by passing the suture close to the limbus through the surface layers of the sclera *(Drawing 16-3)*;

f) when the surface to be repaired is large because of excessive tissue removal, and the classical plastic techniques are problematic, the surgeon should use a free graft of autologous conjunctiva.

COMPLICATIONS WITH PLASTIC SURGERY OF THE CONJUNCTIVA

Excessive removal of conjunctival tissue is a common problem in pterygium surgery, particularly when performed by less experienced surgeons. This event produces a discrepancy between the exposed scleral surface and the insufficient quantity of conjunctiva available to cover it. If the sutures are too tight, dehiscence may be observed in the post-operative with scarring by second intention and unsatisfactory aesthetic results.

Dehiscence is observed in the first week postoperative and is produced by the spontaneous scar retraction of the conjunctiva and the episclera. Treatment consist of peeling back a greater amount of the conjunctival surface and placing small cuts to dissipate the tension of the conjunctival flaps and facilitate the maneuvers of the tissue. A second option is to wait until the conjunctiva has scarred by second intention and then remove the scar tissue. The loss can be repaired by grafting a free flap of conjunctival tissue removed from the supero-temporal quadrant of the same eye. Another complication of the conjunctiva is when it tears or fissures during removal of the pterygium or during the plastic repair.

These conjunctival damages may escape observation or may be considered to have little effect on the final outcome of the operation, but in the days immediately following surgery, this will tend to widen exposing the sclera, like in the dehiscence of the wound line. The treatment of small exposed areas is not necessary, particularly if in a peripheral position; however, if the areas are greater or in a paralimbal position, the treatment is the same as that used for dehiscence of the conjunctiva. Complications of the sclera are unusual or minor; nevertheless the surgeon must pay attention to vigorous diathermy or cauterizations in patients affected by systemic pathologies of collagen tissue as these may thin the tissue or create scleromalacia.

17

TECHNIQUE FOR EXCISION OF THE PTERYGIUM WITHOUT SCLERAL COVER

(Scleral Baring)

INTRODUCTION

Scleral baring is included among the surgical operations where the conjunctival repair is not complete following removal of the pterygium, but the sclera is left exposed for spontaneous repair.

The inspiration of these techniques derives from the theory of "epithelial runs".

In the case of a pterygium, according to this theory, the recurrence is observed when the re-epithelialization of the scleral surface by the surrounding bulbar conjunctiva, takes place before the re-epithelialization of the peri-limbal cornea has been completed.

Following removal of the pterygium, if the conjunctiva is distanced from the limbus, the re-epithelialization of the sclera is delayed but the corneal re-epithelialization continues.

About 3-4 mm of sclera is left uncovered in this technique.

Originally, the techniques for scleral baring were used in the treatment of small primary pterygia; at the time of writing, the major indication is the treatment of evolved or recurrent pterygia but only in association with antimetabolites or beta-irradiation therapy of the scleral surface.

SURGICAL TECHNIQUE

Picò's Technique

- Removal of the head of pterygium and cleaning of the cornea by scraping the corneal surface or with a superficial keratectomy with a dissection spatula.

- Excision of the head of the pterygium as far as the semilunar fold by means of two conjunctival cuts along the edges of the pterygium; the cuts run outwards and are slightly diverging.

- The conjunctiva and the pterygium are peeled from the episcleral adhesions and removed with a vertical cut, which joins the two previous radial cuts, close to the semilunar fold.

- Following the removal of the body, the exposed sclera, is cleaned of fibro-vascular residue and cauterized carefully to leave the surface perfectly clean.

- The upper bulbar conjunctiva is peeled back considerably and cut vertically 3 mm from the limbus for a length of about 1 cm to create a large flap that can be dragged across.

- A Vicryl 7/0 suture is passed through the infero-external angle of the conjunctival flap created and sutured to the edge of the inferior conjunctiva about 3 mm from the limbus. In order to facilitate anchoring the conjunctiva, the more proximal suture runs through the superficial layers of the sclera; at the end of the operation, the conjunctival edge must lie 3-4 mm from the limbus.

Recurrences of about 2% are reported in the treatment of primary pterygium with this technique. However, the aesthetic result is mediocre.

D'Ombrain's Technique

This is a mixed technique that associates scleral baring with the sub-conjunctival excision of the pterygium.

- A fine hook is passed around the limbus to raise the pterygium.

- The pterygium is caught for its entire depth with a toothed forceps; using flat scissors, two slightly diverging incisions are created from the limbus along the edges of the pterygium to reach the semilunar fold.

- The body of the pterygium is peeled from the scleral plane in correspondence to the two incisions so that forceps can be introduced to hold the body steady.

- The apex of the pterygium is scraped with Desmarres knife, and this includes the excision of a thin layer of superficial corneal tissue.

- The detached pterygium is brought close to the medial canthus and gently overturned onto a damp gauze.

- Non-traumatic forceps held by an assistant are used to raise the pterygium; then using non-traumatic straight scissors, the surgeon removes the sub-conjunctival tissue so that the conjunctiva is cleaned of fibro-vascular tissue.

- A small portion of the conjunctiva close to the limbus is removed to leave an exposed area of sclera measuring about 4 mm.

- The remainder of the conjunctiva is distended on the sclera and sutured with silk 6/0 thread.

Compared to the previous technique, this offers a better aesthetic result because more conjunctival tissue is spared. The author recommends that this technique is used in primary pterygium that have not evolved excessively.

Townsend's Technique

- The operation begins with a 0.75 mm pre-corneal incision beyond the head of the pterygium. The head of the pterygium outlined in this way is then dissected to the limbus with a cutting spatula for lamellar keratoplasty. The dissection must involve the layer immediately below Bowman's membrane and the first stromal lamellae.

- The excision of the body occurs through two horizontal incisions, above and below the edges of the body and completed with a vertical cut as far as the internal canthus.

- The sclera is cleaned and the scleral bed is perfectly coagulated.

- Creation of a conjunctival flap in the superior bulbar conjunctiva by means of a vertical incision which starts from the conjunctiva at about 3 mm from the limbus and runs close to the superior fornix. The flap is peeled downwards and sutured to the episclera. At the end of surgery, the conjunctival flap must almost entirely cover the sclera with the exception of the 3 mm behind the limbus.

- In the original technique, at the end of surgery, the tissue was subjected to a 2000 rep dose of beta radiation by means of a Strontium 90 (Sr90) applicator.

Nordan's Technique

- Two 3 mm radial incisions are created in the conjunctiva, starting from the limbus and proceeding along the edges of the body of pterygium.

- Using a blade, two corneal incisions are created around the head of the pterygium close to the limbus which then join the existing conjunctival incisions. The body that has been peeled back and isolated is excised at the medial canthus.

- Following scleral hemostasis and the cleaning of the corneal surface, the remaining conjunctiva, is sutured to the edge of the underlying sclera, leaving a vast area of sclera exposed.

Therapy and Post-Operative Course in the Techniques of Scleral Baring

Post-operative therapy consists of the administration of topical antibiotics (monodose Netilmicin), Artificial tear (sodium hyaluronate) and NSAIDs (if necessary) (Indomethacin eyedrops) to reduce inflammation and pain.

Because of its scar-inhibition action, topical cortisone should be used cautiously and never in the initial 72 hours from surgery, or better still, only following careful clinical evaluation.

Silk sutures in the conjunctiva should be removed after 5-7 days; nylon sutures should be removed after 10-15 days.

18

MITOMYCIN C IN THE TREATMENT OF PTERYGIUM

INTRODUCTION

The use of anti-mitotic drugs to treat pterygia dates back to the Sixties. However, over the years a number of anti-neoplastic drugs have been tested with intra-operative and post-operative treatment protocols. Of all the drugs tested, Mitomycin C is the substance that has produced the best results with fewer side effects and complications.

Yet today, despite the fact that Mitomycin C is generally accepted as the elective anti-mitotic in the surgery of pterygia, the treatment protocols are still a source of discussion and clinical experimentation particularly where the optimal concentration and the duration of treatment are concerned.

PHARMACOLOGICAL CHARACTERISTICS OF MITOMYCIN C

Mitomycin C is an antibiotic isolated from a culture of Streptomyces caespitosus. Its mechanism of action consists of the formation of irreversible bonds between the two chains of DNA, thus preventing cell replication and mitosis.

In the eye, its action inhibits the growth and proliferation of the cells with fibroblastic activity, that in pterygia are responsible for the proliferation of the sub-conjunctival tissue and fibrosis.

Mitomycin is the elective choice over other drugs with a similar mechanism of action because in vitro studies have shown that the inhibitory ac-

tion of Mitomycin C on the fibroblasts of the eye is 2.5 times greater than in the other tissues of the body. A recent study, completed to evaluate the optimal concentration of the drug in the treatment of pterygia, reported that the growth of fibroblasts of pterygia in culture with 0.02% or 0.04% mitomycin was 50% in both groups following five minutes of exposure to the substance.[78,79]

This above fact makes the drug the elective choice in the treatment of neoplasias of the ocular surface.

The drug's ability to inhibit the proliferation of ocular fibroblasts also makes it more dangerous as it can delay or inhibit many repair processes of the ocular tissues.

INDICATIONS FOR THE USE OF MITOMYCIN C

The indications reported in the literature are as follows:
- inflamed primary pterygium, highly vascularized with the cornea involved for at least 1 mm;
- pterygium with previous recurrences;
- pterygium localized in the temporal zone;
- pterygium in risk patients or patients aged below 30 years.

Our indications are as follows:
- primary pterygium Type I in risk patients

- Primary pterygium Type II in patients with relapse in the fellow eye

- Recurrent pterygium Type II with abundant fibro-vascular proliferation

- Recurrent pterygium Type II following failure of a limbal graft.

PREPARATION OF MITOMYCIN C

Commercial product: Mitomycin C powder, 2 mg, 10 mg 20 mg.

Solvent: BSS for intraoperative chemical use (Biotech).

TREATMENT PROTOCOLS

In 1964, the first positive results from using Mitomycin C were reported with a concentration of 0.04%, administered following the surgical removal of pterygium.

Subsequently, many scientific studies and papers confirmed the positive results using different treatment protocols and different concentrations.

Intraoperative Treatment

This is associated with a surgical technique of scleral baring. Mitomycin C is applied to the sclera behind the limbus by means of a sponge soaked in 0.02%-0.04% Mitomycin.

There must be continuous contact with the sclera for 3-5 minutes.

The most popular protocol, even from our own experience, is the intraoperative application of 0.02% Mitomycin for five minutes.

- Once the pterygium has been removed using scleral baring, the sclera around the limbus is exposed

- A sponge measuring 5x5 mm is soaked in a 0.02% solution of Mitomycin C.

- The sponge is applied to the bare sclera and kept in position for 3-5 minutes (or for the time stated in the chosen protocol)

- Following treatment the scleral surface is washed continually for at least 5 minutes with a saline solution.

Post-Operative Protocols

There are a number of protocols for the post-operative treatment with Mitomycin C but there are no precise indications available.

The concentrations vary between 0.01% and 0.1% and the number of applications varies between 2-4 per day for between 5-14 days.

TABLE SUMMARIZING THE POST-OPERATIVE PROTOCOLS WITH MITOMYCIN C			
	Concentration	No. Applications	Duration of therapy
Protocol No. 1[92]	0.01%	2 times/day	5 days
Protocol No. 2[93,86,88,92]	0.02%	2 times/day	5 days
Protocol No. 3[94]	0.04%	3 times/day	3 days
Protocol No. 4[95]	0.04%	3 times/day	7 days
Protocol No. 5[93]	0.04%	4 times/day	14 days
Protocol No. 6[87]	0.04%	4 times/day	14 days
Protocol No. 7[84]	0.05%	4 times/day	14 days

TABLE SUMMARIZING THE RESULTS OF TREATMENT WITH MITOMYCIN REPORTED IN THE LITERATURE						
Author	**Type of operation**	**Use of Mito-C**	**No. patients**	**Follow-up**	**% relapses**	**Protocol for Mitomycin C**
Hayasaka	exp. sclera	post-op	99	3-8 years	7-11%	0.02/0.04% 2 times/day 5-7 days
Singh	exp. sclera	post-op	62	23 weeks	2.2%	0.04% 4 times/day 14 days
Rosenthal	exp. sclera	post-op	70	1 year	5%	0.02% 2 times/day 5 days
Mahar	excision	post-op	17	13-19 months	0%	0.04% 4 times/day 14 days
Mastropasqua	exp. sclera	intraop.	30	7-30 months	6.6%	0.04% for 3 minutes
Frucht-Pery	exp. sclera	intraop	40	6-15 months	5%	0.02% for 5 minutes
Frucht-Pery	exp. sclera	post-op.	75	7-27 months	8%	0.01-0.02% 5 times/day 5 days
Cano-Parra	excision	intra-op	66	12-23 months	3.33%	0.01% for 5 minutes
Rachmiel	exp. sclera	post-op.	38	6-11 months	2.6%	0.02% 2 times a day for 5 days
Chen PP	exp. sclera	post-op	24	6-22 months	38%	0.02% 2 times a day for 5 days
Frucht-Pery	exp. sclera	intraop	81	12-28 months	4%	0.02% for 5 minutes
Anduze	sub-conj inj	intraop	135	10 mths-3 years	1.5%	Subconj inj 0.05-0.1 ml at 0.05%
Helal	exp. sclera	intraop	156	11 months	5.75%	0.01% for 3 minutes

Results from the Treatment With Mitomycin C

The reports from using the intraoperative protocols show recurrences of between 1.5-6%, with a minimum follow-up of 12 months.[79,80,81,82,83,84]

With the post-operative protocols, the number of recurrences varied considerably, between 0-38%.[84,85,86,87,88]

Complications Deriving from the Use of Mitomycin C

The literature reports numerous mild complications and transitory complications deriving from the use of Mitomycin C in the treatment of pterygium; other more serious complications have also been reported which may lead to the functional and anatomic loss of the eye.

For this reason, the routine use of Mitomycin C in the treatment of pterygium must be handled with extreme care *(Figure 18-1)*.

A delay in corneal re-epithelialization is considered to be a complication, or more correctly, this is the side effect that is observed with major frequency.

The epithelial damage is non-specific and is observed as a punctate keratitis; thinned zones and corneal dellen are also observed around the treatment zone.

Less frequently episcleral granulomas are observed and are generally small in size.

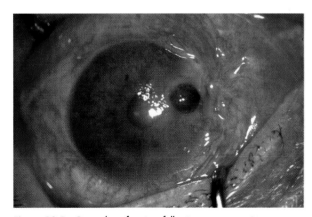

Figure 18-1. *Corneal perforation following post-operative treatment with Mitomycin C. About 2 weeks after the end of treatment, the patient is affected by a marginal corneal ulcer that has progressed as far as the corneal perforation.*

With the intraoperative use serious complications are unusual; with the post-operative protocols however, necrosis of the sclera, glaucoma and cataract have been reported.[85,89,90]

The complications can be directly or indirectly attributed to Mitomycin's inhibition of the repair processes.

The more important complications are:

- corneal and scleral ulcers (to the degree of perforation);

- calcific plaques on the sclera;

- pyogenic granulomas;

- secondary glaucoma;

- cataract;

- anterior uveitis.

Necrosis of the sclera, following the post-operative use of Mitomycin, has been observed even two years from treatment,[91] suggesting that the control visits would be continued for a longer period when Mitomycin has been used.

19

Other Surgical Techniques Used in Pterygium

Amniotic Membrane Graft

The use of the amniotic membrane in ocular surgery dates back to the Forties[99,100] and the very first report of its use in pterygium surgery was reported by Panzardi in the Sixties (1964). This author reported outstanding aesthetic and therapeutic results in small pterygia while he made no reference to the results in the evolved or recurrent forms.

Anatomically, the amniotic membrane coats the inside of the amniotic sac and consists of a thin layer of collagen covered with mono-stratified epithelium resting on a basement membrane.

The amniotic membrane has some interesting biological properties. It is anti-adhesive, anti-bacterial, provides wound protection, pain relief and encourages epithelial growth.[101,102,103,104]

However, the most important factor is the absence of immune reaction that allows it to be used with no antigen incompatibility.

The basement membrane of the amniotic membrane contains Type IV collagen and laminine similar to the basement membrane of the conjunctiva.

This makes it an ideal graft material of the conjunctival basement membrane and an excellent substrate for the growth of the epithelial cells.

The epithelium of the amniotic membrane actually secretes growth factors: the basic fibroblast growth factor, hepatocyte growth factor and transforming growth factor and other factors that encourage the differentiation and proliferation of the conjunctival and corneal epithelium.

Removal and Preservation of the Amniotic Membrane

There is no standard protocol regarding the removal technique and the preservation of the amniotic membrane.

The greatest problem is the tissue source that requires a good organizational interface with the maternity units that supply the tissue.

The donor patient must be negative for all potentially transmissible viral infections (the protocol used for donor corneas can be applied).

The removal must take place in aseptic conditions and consists of the separation, by dissection, of the amniotic membrane from the underlying placenta chorion.

Once the membrane has been removed, it is cut into pieces measuring 5x5 mm; it is washed abundantly with an antibiotic solution (gentamycin 1 mg /ml or alternately with streptomycin 50mg/ml and sodium penicillin 50 mg/ml) and then washed abundantly with 0.01 M PBS or sterile saline solution.

After the epithelial face has been marked, the pieces of amniotic membrane are placed on a sponge support and then transferred to a storage container for preservation.

Storage at -80°C would appear to be the best system for conserving the vitality of the amniotic membrane; this allows the epithelial cells to survive for up to 70 days of storage.[105]

In our own experience we have observed good preservation for up to three weeks in a medium at +4°C. This solution is also more practical, though microbiologically less efficacious than the storage at -80°C. Colonies of mycetes or bacteria may form and these can be observed as a change in the color and the transparency of the medium.

Indications for the Graft of Amniotic Membrane

Amniotic membrane has been used in the past for the treatment of skin ulcers in severe burns, in the skin ulcers of the Stevens-Johnson syndrome and pelvic and vaginal surgery. In ophthalmology, it has been used in the treatment of cicatricial pemphigoid, in the treatment of burns to the eye surface and in the treatment of persisting epithelial defects.

The use of the amniotic membrane in pterygium surgery, to replace the missing conjunctiva, has not produced excellent results; in the recurrent and evolved forms, recurrences have been reported in about 40% of these cases, and an incidence of 10% in primary pterygia.[109]

The amniotic membrane used to repair large eye surfaces is very interesting; in these cases an autologous graft of limbal conjunctiva must be associated to supply epithelial cells to the membrane to be colonized.

This method is used today in the treatment of sub-conjunctiva fibrosis of repeatedly recurrent pterygia where the proliferation of abundant sub-conjunctival fibrous tissue causes scar symblepharon at the fornices, ectropion of the lacrimal duct and diplopia because of the involvement of the tendon of the medial rectus muscle. These are clinical forms where previous excision surgery stimulated fibrous tissue growth[110] *(Figure 19-1)*.

Various surgical techniques have been used to treat fibrosis - lamellar keratoplasty, grafts of autologous conjunctiva, grafts of limbal conjunctiva - but to date none has demonstrated real efficacy in

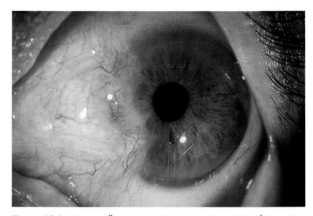

Figure 19-1. *Repeatedly recurrent Pterygium Type II. In this patient, following numerous operations of simple excision and recurrence, there is the marked proliferation of sub-conjunctival fibrous tissue which caused an infiltration to the tendon of the medial rectus muscle with diplopia in lateral vision and a deficit in abduction. With this complication, a graft of amniotic membrane can be considered.*

blocking the growth of the sub-conjunctival fibrous tissue;[106,107,108] the anti-metabolites (Mitomycin C) and beta therapy despite being powerful inhibitors of fibro-vascular proliferation, can cause a series of complications to the cornea and the sclera.

Surgical Procedure for the Amniotic Membrane Graft

- After having removed the head of pterygium from the cornea, and once the surface keratectomy has been completed, all the sub-conjunctival fibrous tissue is removed until the sclera is exposed. This must be done very carefully at the medial canthus to avoid damaging the tendon of the medial rectus muscle.

- The amniotic membrane is removed from its container and is placed on a support of porous material, and washed abundantly with antibiotic and saline solutions.

- The membrane is placed on the exposed sclera with the epithelium facing upwards; it is fixed in position with nylon 9/0 or 10/0 sutures. The epithelial face can be identified easily if it was marked earlier or alternately, it can be identified as the face that was not adhered to the placenta chorion.

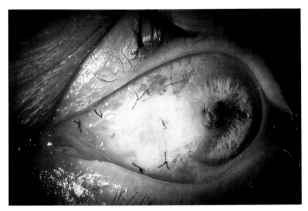

Figure 19-2. *Graft of a flap of amniotic membrane in a patient with repeatedly recurrent pterygium and sub-conjunctival fibrosis.*

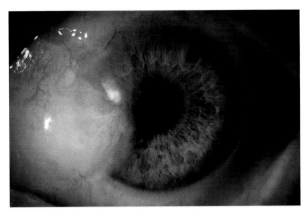

Figure 19-3. *A graft of buccal mucosa. This patient is also shown in Figure 19-2 where the pterygium recurred just a few months after the graft with amniotic membrane. The graft of buccal mucosa resolved the problem of diplopia, but the buccal mucosa showed evident post-operative hypertrophy with obvious aesthetic problems.*

- The flap of limbal conjunctiva is removed from the superior part as previously described, removing a small flap of cornea.

- The flap of limbal conjunctiva is placed 1-2 mm from the nasal limbus and sutured into position with interrupted sutures in nylon 9/0 or 10/0. The suture points must pass through the full depth of the flap, the underlying amniotic membrane and the superficial layers of the sclera *(Figure 19-2)*.

Buccal Mucosal Graft

For many years, Rollet's technique was considered to be highly efficacious in the prevention of recurrences of pterygium. At the time of writing, it has been replaced with autologous conjunctival grafts and other "barrier" techniques. The technique consists of grafting a large flap of buccal mucosa (measuring 10 mm x 15 mm) at the limbus following removal of the pterygium.

However, in order to achieve good results, the author stresses the importance of grafting a thin flap, free from sub-mucosal tissue.

Despite the good results in the recurrences, the aesthetic results with this technique are poor because of the different color of the buccal mucosa compared to the surrounding conjunctiva.[80]

The buccal mucosa is still being used today for the repair of large surfaces of scleral that were bared during the removal of the pterygium *(Figure 19-3)*.

The main indication of this technique is in the case of recurrent pterygia with sub-conjunctival fibrosis that produces symblepharon, epiphora and restriction of abduction, in those cases when no amniotic membrane is available and it is not possible to use a graft of autologous conjunctiva.

Removal Technique

- The lower lip is turned over and outwards and the sampling area is infiltrated with local anesthesia;

- The flap is measured with a compass (length and width) and the buccal mucosa is cut with scalpel.

- The mucosa is subjected to mild traction with forceps; scissors are used to separate the submucosa progressively over the entire area outlined.

- The flap created is placed on a wet gauze and washed abundantly with an antibiotic solution.

- The sample site is coagulated or compressed between two fingers to reduce bleeding. It is then sutured with absorbable sutures and silk 6/0.

- The flap is overturned with the epithelial surface facing downwards. It is held on the hand and scissors are again used to remove the layer of sub-mucosal tissue and the minor salivary glands. Following this step, the flap appears to be thin and semi-transparent.

- The flap is positioned on the sclera and sutured with interrupted sutures using the method applied for the conjunctival grafts.

Post-Operative Course and Complications

In the first week following the amniotic membrane graft, there is complete re-epithelialization of the cornea and the colonization of the amniotic membrane; there is a considerable improvement in the conditions of the fornices and a reduction or disappearance of diplopia. Few complications are reported in the literature and are of little importance; they include pyogenic granuloma, areas of scleral thinning, dellen; the incidence of complications do not differ from the percentages reported with other techniques of mucosa grafting. The complications with this type of surgery include:

• Infection

This is a rare occurrence but can jeopardize the vitality of the graft tissue with consequent re-absorption of the tissue through enzymatic lysis by the bacteria.

• Hemorrhage

This may be observed early in the post-operative period and involve the episcleral space. This situation may cause the graft tissue to rise up and prevent its attachment. Mild bleeding under the flap does not cause any particular problems. This latter complication is frequent when the hemostasis of the scleral bed has not been completed as carefully and precisely as it should have been.

• Necrosis of the flap

This complication involves the buccal grafts and can appear because of:
- excessive manipulation of the flap during removal or grafting;
- inadequate preparation of the receiving bed;
- inadequate fixing of the graft tissue;
- infection.

A necrotic flap is white and opaque, it lacks blood vessels or is crossed with fine capillaries that tend to "whiten" in a matter of days.

When necrosis is advanced or total, the graft must be removed and replaced; if necrosis is partial, the surgeon can attempt to improve the vascularization by applying warm wet compresses and vasodilatory eyedrops.

• Pyogenic granuloma

This is caused by inadequate suturing of the conjunctiva or an inflammatory reaction to the suture. It is encouraged by introflexion of the conjunctival suture line *(Figure 19-4)*.

• Epithelial cysts

These can form when epithelial cells persist under the graft.

• Perforation of the conjunctiva

A hole in the conjunctival flap tends to widen under the effects of physiological retraction of the tissue and decreases the effects of surgery.

• Dislocation of the graft

In the event of inadequate fixation or sutures that are under excessive tension, retraction or detachment of the graft may be observed. It will tend to withdraw exposing the underlying sclera.

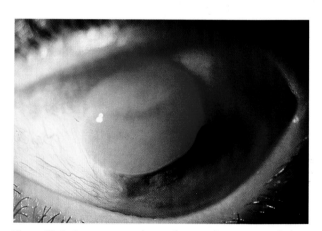

Figure 19-4. *Pyogenic granuloma. The granuloma appeared about three weeks after the graft of a buccal mucosa flap. This complication must be treated surgically.*

• Irregularity of the mucous graft and retraction of the caruncle

This is a late complication that may produce very poor aesthetic results.

When the repair of the conjunctival loss is performed using labial mucosa, folds may form in the mucosa at the medial canthus with different colored zones compared to the surrounding conjunctiva.

In these cases, when we are certain there is no recurrence, the mucosa can be shifted from its medial position to a "hidden" conjunctival zone and the conjunctiva of this zone grafted at the medial canthus.

During this plastic surgery graft of the conjunctiva, the sclera must be bared and all the fibrovascular tissue eliminated.

On other occasions, there may be a horizontal fold in the conjunctiva and in the sub-conjunctival tissue which resembles the body of a pterygium but which lacks the clinical characteristics of progression.

In these pterygoid forms, it is also possible to perform a graft of autologous from the same or the fellow eye.

RESULTS

Following the graft of a flap of amniotic membrane, the reported recurrences lie between 10% for the primary forms and 37% for the recurrent forms.[109] These percentages refer to the simple graft, a procedure that is not widely used. The use of the amniotic membrane would appear to be extremely interesting when associated with a graft of limbal conjunctiva in the treatment of sub-conjunctival fibrosis in repeatedly recurrent pterygia. The problems linked to the tissue supplies and its storage prevent the dissemination of this technique.

The use of buccal mucosa still has some indications in those centers where amniotic membrane is not available and in the cases where it is not possible to remove autologous conjunctiva.

The association of lamellar keratoplasty with a graft of buccal mucosa can provide excellent results in severely advanced pterygia, though the aesthetic results are less than satisfactory.

Long-term studies have not been performed on the results with an isolated limbal graft or the graft used in association with the amniotic membrane as a substrate.

20

PRINCIPLES OF OPERATING TECHNIQUES FOR PTERYGIUM

REMOVAL OF THE HEAD OF THE PTERYGIUM

The head of the pterygium consists of two anatomical layers which have different consistencies and which behave differently during excision.

The superficial layer consists of a thin conjunctival layer, that adheres to a mobile relaxed tissue of the underlying plane.

The deeper sub-conjunctival or pre-corneal layer is firmly attached to the superficial layers of the cornea.

In ocular surgery, the precise resection to remove the mobile tissue, for example the superficial layer of the head of a pterygium, proves difficult because of the mobility of the tissue.

This low "cutability" is an important protective feature against accidental damage to the cornea and to the conjunctiva itself.

The excision of the adhered tissue, for example in the deep pre-corneal resection of the head of pterygium, allows more precise surgical maneuvers but does not offer the same amount of protection as the relaxed tissue does.

As a result, involuntary damage to the cornea is more frequent (*Drawings 20-1, 20-2*).

The removal of the head of the pterygium from the cornea can be performed using various types of instruments: blades, cutting spatulas or scissors.

In removal with scissors, if the cut is made in the superficial mobile layer, it will not reach the adhesion plane with the cornea and a large portion of the tissue will not be removed, but if the head is pulled using forceps, the cut will be improved and the surgeon can reach as far as the attachment to the fixed part that is adhered to the cornea.

Avulsion of the pterygium works according to the same principles; the tension created with strong forceps is sufficient to separate the mobile portion from the adhered part and can even detach the tissue from the corneal cleavage plane.

The removal of the head with cutting instruments, blades or spatulas, follows different rules.

When the tip of the blade penetrates the apex of the pterygium, the dissection is in the layer of sub-epithelial fibers of the cornea; however, if the tip enters 1-1.5 mm in front of the apex, the dissection will be deeper, in the cleavage plane with the superficial stromal lamellae.

The surgeon should be familiar with these concepts.

On the basis of the surgical program, if a keratectomy is necessary the surgeon must be able to decide whether the dissection must start in front of the apex.

However, if this is not considered important, or if trephination has been planned later, he must decide whether the dissection can be started at the apex of the pterygium.

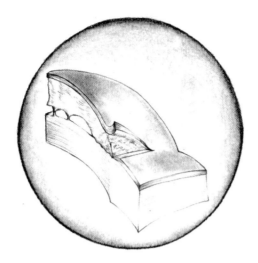

Drawing 20-1. *The drawing shows the thin superficial layer and its relationship with the relaxed tissue below.*

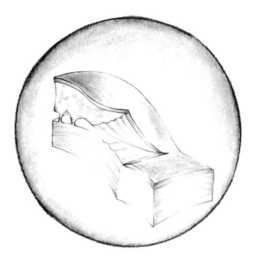

Drawing 20-2. *The drawing shows a deep pre-corneal dissection. The adhesion of the cornea allows a precise resection of the tissue but facilitates accidental damage to the cornea such as irregular keratectomy, illustrated in the drawing.*

EXCISION OF THE BODY

Like the head, the body of the pterygium consists of two anatomical layers: a superficial layer of conjunctival mucosa and a deeper episcleral layer. Again for the body, the dissection of these two layers is different and can be classified as superficial or deep dissection.

The superficial dissection separates the layer of conjunctival mucosa from the fibro-vascular tissue while the deep dissection provides access to the scleral surface.

The highly relaxed episcleral space is easily accessible in ocular surgery contrary to the situation with the virtual sub-conjunctival space that is firmly adhered.

The deep episcleral dissection can therefore be done with blunt instruments and this easily separates the adhesions with the scleral surface.

In some pathological situations (conjunctival scars, sub-conjunctival fibrosis) the adhesion with the sclera is greater and the episcleral space is less accessible.

Infiltrating this space with a liquid (anesthetic or saline solution) to create tension in the episcleral tissue makes it easy for the surgeon to identify the space and proceed with the dissection.

Deep episcleral excision is used to remove the full depth of the body of the pterygium *(Drawing 20-3).*

The body of the pterygium is excised from the limbus as far as the semilunar fold and must reach the surface of the sclera to allow the removal of all the fibro-vascular tissue.

Scissors are used for the complete excision of the body.

The correct position of the blade is in continual contact with the sclera, and parallel to it and pushed against its surface.

This will ensure a uniform dissection and will prevent damage to the surrounding anatomical structures (for example, damage to the tendons of the extra-ocular muscles).

Superficial excision to separate the mucosal layer from the sub-conjunctival tissue is used in the selective removal of the sub-mucosal fibro-vascular tissue and separates the fibro-vascular tissue from the conjunctiva without damaging it *(Drawing 20-4).*

The technical difficulties inherent to the selective removal of the fibro-vascular tissue are undoubtedly greater and related to the difficulty involved in separating a serrated and invisible plane that is defined by the surgeon himself as he pro-

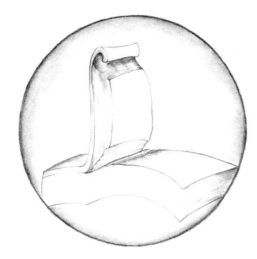

Drawing 20-3. *The drawing shows a full-depth excision of the pterygium.*

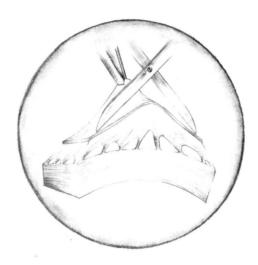

Drawing 20-5. *Deep conjunctival dissection. The drawing shows the wide opening of the scissors.*

ceeds with the dissection; the size, the mobility, the transparency and the thinness of the conjunctival flap depend on the surgeon's ability to accurately separate the sub-epithelial fibers.

The separation of the conjunctival layer from the sub-epithelial fibers proves difficult because of the poor "cutability" of these fibers.

During the dissection, they will move up or down causing a deviation in the cut direction. Some measures can be taken to increase the "cutability"

of the sub-epithelial fibers and reduce their tendency to slide.

Cutability can be increased by holding the fibers with forceps or the scissors, however, the tension will be positive only if the fibers are firmly adhered to the underlying sclera, otherwise a thin flap cannot be cut. This will not be eliminated even if the upward traction exerted is stronger, because only the fibers towards the epithelium will be pulled producing an even thicker flap.

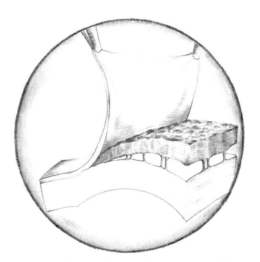

Drawing 20-4. *The drawing shows a selective excision of the conjunctival layer from the fibro-vascular layer of the body of the pterygium.*

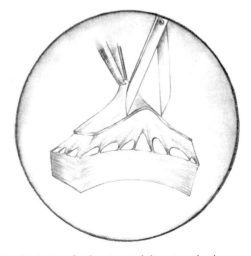

Drawing 20-6. *Superficial conjunctival dissection. The drawing shows the position of the scissors which "nip" the tissue.*

When the surgeon performs a superficial dissection, his primary objective is to conserve the existing deep attachment points and create other new ones; he must avoid opening the episcleral space or infiltrating the space with liquids or anesthetics.

The choice of surgical instruments is also very important in the choice of the dissection type; for example, the scissors are guided in the deep episcleral dissection with a large opening, whereas in the superficial dissection, the opening must be minimal; in the deep dissection, the surgeon uses blunt scissors, in the superficial dissection, sharp, pointed scissors must be used to nip the tissue *(Drawings 20-5, 20-6)*.

In conclusion, the same rules for the superficial dissection apply to the surgery of the free mucosal flaps where thin flaps that are free from episcleral tissue improve the therapeutic and aesthetic result of the operation.

Suture of the Conjunctiva

Suturing the conjunctiva must follow a series of precise rules. The edges of the conjunctival wounds have a natural tendency to retract and wrinkle due to the presence of elastic sub-epithelial fibers *(Drawing 20-3)*.

When it is necessary to mobilize and close the edges of the conjunctival wound, the physiological retraction must be counter-balanced with counter-traction; the fibers are held steady with the teeth of conjunctival forceps and only then stretched to be closed and sutured. This maneuver allows the surface epithelial layer to expand and be perforated with a suture needle at the edge of conjunctiva. The intrinsic malleability of the conjunctival tissue provides a wide range of choice in terms of suture technique and the material used, because only on very rare occasions do the deformations of the tissue caused by the suture compromise the outcome of the operation.

Once sutured, the conjunctiva has excellent post-operative adhesion to the underlying layers but only if this occurs on a vascularized substrate, whereas it is poor on the smooth epithelialized corneal surface or on a sclera that has been bared and cleaned. This is why, in order to adhere better, free conjunctival flaps used in the surgery of pterygium must be fixed to vascularized tissue in the surrounding conjunctiva, or anchored by a couple of sutures that pass through the surface layers of the sclera.

Keratectomy in Pterygium

The external fibrous sheath of the eye consists of layered, lamellar tissue. The lamellae are uniform in the cornea and have a precise shape; in the sclera, they become disordered and irregular. The anatomical difference can be correlated with different surgical characteristics related to the dissection. All the maneuvers of the dissection are influenced by the intraocular pressure. Those surgical techniques that are efficacious with a normal or higher-than-normal ocular pressure will not be successful under conditions of lower-than-normal pressure, and vice-versa.

Manipulations that have the same purpose must be planned for before or after the globe has been opened. The corneal and scleral tissue behave differently if cut with scissors or a trephine under conditions of higher or lower ocular pressure. The normal or hypertonic globe can be easily immobilized with forceps even at a point distant from the cutting instrument and this will permit a more precise, regular dissection.

Under conditions of low intraocular pressure, it is difficult to fix the globe and the manipulations can be efficacious only if the tissue is caught and immobilized very close to the cutting edge of the instrument. This difficulty will naturally influence the precision of the cut and the dissection.

The incision of the cornea with a blade positioned obliquely to the corneal surface will tend to remain on a single trajectory and on the same plane if the intraocular pressure is normal or higher-than-normal; however, if the pressure is low, there will be considerable downward deflection of the laminae and the dissection will be deeper. As it is not easy to evaluate the possible lamellar deflection, there is the risk of poor precision when oblique incisions are performed. In lamellar keratectomies that require enormous precision, initially, the incisions must be perpendicular to the lamellae to then proceed parallel to them; the vertical incision defines the depth of the cut while the parallel dissection defines the width of the cut and the uniformity of the keratectomy.

The objective of trephining and the keratectomy is to obtain and maintain the chosen cleavage plane. The depth of a small corneal incision can be estimated by the amount of blade immersed in the cut tissue; for longer or circular incisions, it is easier to maintain the depth by blocking the blade with a specific device (such as the internal block in a trephine, the feet of the refractive surgery blades or by using pre-calibrated instruments). These devices work only if the blade is held perpendicularly at a right angle (90°) to the tissue surface. The preset depth will never be achieved along the entire cut line and the difference in the cut depth depends on the shape of the blade and its orientation.

In the initial stages of a keratectomy, in the cornea at a pre-set depth from the cleavage plane, the surgeon must create sufficient space for the introduction of a cutting spatula which can rotate for at least 90° with respect to the entrance point, permitting the lamellar dissection.

To evaluate the depth of the keratectomy, the edge of the incision can be caught with forceps and pulled upwards; the tissue will lengthen and this will give the surgeon a precise evaluation of the depth. In a layered tissue such as the cornea, the resistance of the cutting edge during the incision diminishes in the direction of the lamellae but increases in a direction perpendicular to them. What results is an incision that is progressively deviated on a route parallel to the direction of the corneal lamellae, the so-called lamellar deviation. The surgeon can intervene on the lamellar deviation by using very sharp/clean-cutting instruments (clean-cutting is the ability to divide a tissue with a blade) and regulating the direction and the speed of the blade movements on the tissue being cut. A direction parallel to the blade edge will increase precision.

Lamellar deviation will be encouraged if the blades do not produce a clean cut; this may be advantageous during the dissection of the layers but is a disadvantage when the lamellae have to be cut in section.

In both half-moon peripheral, and large and circular keratectomies for pterygium, the cut is achieved with curved incisions, first using a trephine and then by hand using a cutting spatula. Trephining produces a perpendicular section of lamellae that do not have the same spatial orientation; as a result, there is a high probability that the cut will be deviated. In the creation of a cleavage plane, the surgeon uses pointed cutting instruments that will reduce the lateral resistance of the tissue during penetration thus increasing the precision of the cut.

Another technical hint to improve the precision of the cut is to place the cutting instrument vertically at the base of the groove and then push it laterally while maintaining the vertical position. In lamellar keratoplasty, the creation of a cleavage plane occurs within a very small space in a very thin corneal incision and for this reason a short, angled blade such as a Paufique spatula is ideal. It facilitates the entrance to one of the corneal planes, and creates a precise, uniform cleavage plane.

Keratectomy can be performed in a number of ways that differ through the way the corneal flap is sliced and the interlamellar fibers are divided.

We can identify three methods:

a. with the flap in situ

b. with the flap raised

c. with the flap displaced

In the keratectomy with the flap in situ, the fibers and the lamellae are split while keeping the flap in its anatomical position *(Drawing 20-7)*.

With this technique, there is no deformation of the fibers during dissection if the blade has a curvature similar to that of the corneal surface. However, there is minimal deformation with a right-angled blade.

The interlamellar fibers to be split maintain their natural position and their tension depends on the thickness of the blade. The dissection of a flap in situ is difficult to control visually but is ideal in those cases where the dissection can be performed rapidly as the fibers to be split are hidden by the superimposed flap and can be evaluated only by interpreting the position of the blade.

The blade can be viewed directly when the cor-

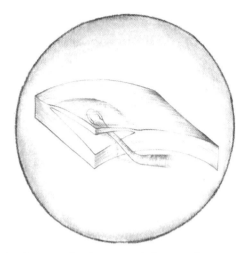

Drawing 20-7. *Lamellar dissection with the in situ flap.*

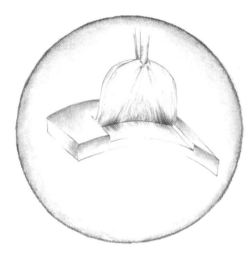

Drawing 20-8. *Lamellar dissection with the flap under tension.*

nea is transparent but in opaque tissue it can be controlled only indirectly by raising the blade slightly to produce a bump that is visible of the outside of the tissue surface.

In the dissection with the flap raised or displaced, there is a direct view of the dissection point and the fibers can be cut with greater precision. With these techniques, the difficulties arise because the fibers are subjected to deforming forces that create folds at the hinge.

The surgeon should know about how these deformations on the hinge arise so that he can avoid performing irregular dissections because of a change of cleavage plane. When the flap is raised, the lateral edges are raised and stretched and the fibers in this area are under tension, while at the center of the flap, as this is depressed, the fibers appear to be more relaxed *(Drawing 20-8)*. This means that the blade will cut or separate deeper stromal fibers at the edge of the hinge and more superficial fibers at the center.

Another effect is that the cutability of the more peripheral fibers is greater than the less distended, more central fibers. As a result there is a greater probability that the dissection plane will be modified in the peripheral part of the hinge compared to the central part.

The effects of the folds can be reduced by shortening the length of the hinge; this can be done by dissecting the peripheral fibers first followed by the more central ones, and if possible, subdividing the flap into smaller segments. In this way the hinge becomes shorter and the central fibers are gradually subjected to greater tension.

In the displaced flap *(Drawing 20-9)*, the tension in the interlamellar fibers does not depend on the traction exerted by the forceps but on the quantity and the degree of tension in the displaced flap. We can state that in a displaced flap, the tension in the interlamellar fibers is uniform for the length of the hinge and the dissection can be more uniform. The thickness of the flap is the factor that has a greater influence on the tension in the hinge; thinner flaps, which can be deformed more easily, create less tension on the hinge, and uneven tension develops only if there is considerable resistance to folding along the axis of the hinge in thicker flaps.

Uniform tension can be maintained as the flap is being created and independent of its length. This characteristic permits easier dissection and more uniform thickness if compared to the other methods.

When compared to the flap in situ, dissection of the raised or displaced flap provides a much clearer view of the interlamellar fibers. So when a clean dissection is required, both techniques can be used.

Summarizing, in order to have a more precise

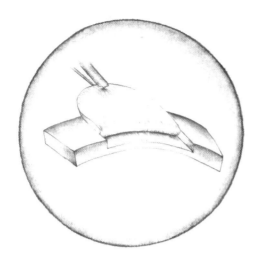

Drawing 20-9. *Lamellar dissection with the flap to one side.*

dissection, the position of the flap must be changed so that, if necessary, the tension in the interlamellar fibers of the hinge can be varied. In relation to the manual technique, this is performed by changing the direction of the dissection, or rather by changing the direction and the movement of the blade. In the raised flap, the fibers are pulled upwards and by cutting them at the lower end, we obtain a thicker flap; as a result, the thickness of the flap can be changed by the vertical movements of the blade. In the displaced flap, the exposed fibers assume a more horizontal orientation and the thickness of the flap can be changed by the horizontal movements of the blade.

TREPHINATION

The trephines are circular blades that cut or remove circular pieces of tissue of pre-determined shape and diameter. In theory, a trephine will remove identical discs from different eyes and this absolute congruity is of great importance in a corneal transplant, as the discrepancies between the donor and recipient corneas will generate deformation of the flap and astigmatism. In actual fact, each trephination has individual variations that produce slightly different shapes and diameters.

The discrepancies are caused by the displace-

ment of the blade in the tissue and are caused by asymmetrical resistance in the tissue; the greatest discrepancies are observed when the incision is started with the trephine and terminated with other instruments. Trephination done with hand trephines is also conditioned by the diameter of the hand-piece and the excursion of the cut. The circumference of the hand-piece determines the number of rotations made by the trephine rotated between the fingers; the greater the diameter of the hand-piece, the smaller the number of rotations between the fingers and vice-versa. Therefore, trephines with smaller hand-piece diameters have a greater trephining action.

The use of a trephine with a central piston used for less-than-full-length corneal trephination - as in lamellar keratoplasty - allows the exclusion of variables linked to the initial penetration of the anterior chamber; tissue more difficult to cut, unequal distribution of the resistance along the circumference of the blade and elimination of the rotation of the split portion of the corneal disc towards the portion that has not yet been penetrated.

The trephining movement can be split into two vectors: push the component perpendicular to the surface; and rotation parallel to the tissue surface.

The push vector deepens the cut while the rotation vector creates an action of traction that increases the "cleanness" of the cut procedure. The resistance to trephination depends on where the trephine drill comes into contact with the tissue, and this changes with the penetration depth.

The balance between the forces and the resistances is such that the action of the trephine is different on the disc of corneal tissue and on the surrounding cornea. In trephination with LK, the resistance is distributed uniformly along the circumference of the blade because the initial resistance depends on the resistance of the cutting edge. In the deepening phase, the lateral resistance increases and this contributes to stabilizing the tracks of the trephine; proceeding with the trephination process, the precision of the incision improves and the extension of the cutting movement can gradually be increased, increasing the number of revolutions of the trephine hand-piece between the fingers.

The high lateral resistance offered by the tissue means that the manual trephines can also be guided with precision. Because of the high lateral resistance, once the operator has started the trephination, he is unable to change the cutting direction as the result depends entirely on the characteristics of the cut inherent to the instrument. In the push systems, the lateral resistance is asymmetrical and the lamellar deflection can displace the tissue towards the trephine aperture; the degree of the deflection depends on the intraocular pressure (low "cutability" of the tissue). Under equal conditions, equal intraocular pressure in the donor and recipient eyes should produce identical corneal discs. Lamellar deflection can be minimized by reducing the push vector, applying moderate pressure on the trephine and completing the cut largely through rotation and not through pressure.

21

FINAL COMMENTS

Our experience in the treatment of pterygia revolves largely around lamellar keratoplasty and surgery with autologous conjunctival grafts or grafts of other mucous tissue.

Our current experiments with grafts of autologous stem cells from the limbus and the use of amniotic membrane would appear to confirm that a pterygium probably derives from damage to the stem cells of the nasal limbus; as a result the most physiological therapy must involve techniques that fully restore the physiology in this region.

The preliminary clinical results are very positive, the complications are absent and recurrences are very rare. If this trend is confirmed, we predict a considerable reduction or total disappearance of pterygia Type III and possibly a re-examination of the treatment for pterygium Type I.

At the time of writing, our behavior with pterygia can be described as cautious; we intervene only when there are valid reasons or when the pterygium show evident clinical signs of evolution.

Undoubtedly, pterygium Type II is the most common clinical form, with more heterogeneous clinical features, and creates greater problems in terms of the choice of surgery.

Our preference at the moment lies with the barrier techniques with the autologous grafts of limbal conjunctiva and the half-moon peripheral keratoplasty.

In pterygium Type III, wide or total manual lamellar keratoplasty is still the most suitable technique, despite the fact that problems linked to the interface condition the visual results. *Drawing 21-1* illustrates most of the surgery used in evolved pterygium: limbal grafts, peripheral or central lamellar keratoplasty for optical objective.

We are also beginning to see a large number of techniques for the treatment of pterygia:, the treatments of the optical zone using the excimer laser or with mechanized lamellar keratoplasty.

One very interesting development that we feel has an enormous potential for the future is the use of the amniotic membrane. In addition to treating the sub-conjunctival fibrosis, the amniotic membrane would appear to provide the ideal substrate for colonizing the cells of the eye surface.

If studies on the pathophysiology of the limbus show an active role of the stem cells in the pathogenesis of pterygium, a graft of stem cells on a substrate of amniotic membrane may be considered as the etiological treatment of pterygia and result in the disappearance of the recurrences.

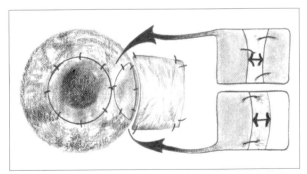

Drawing 21-1. *Examples of limbal and corneal surgery techniques in pterygia.*

BIBLIOGRAPHY

1. Rosenthal JW. Chronology of pterygium therapy. *Am J Ophthalmol* 1953;36:1016-16.

2. Peckar CO. The aetiology and histo-pathogenesis of pterygium. A review of the literature and a hypothesis. *Doc Ophthalmol* 1972;31:141-157.

3. Scarpa A., Rognetta. Du ptérygion. In: Traité pratique des maladies qui affectent ces organes. In: Bayle M, et al. *Encyclopédie des sciences médicales; ou traité general, methodique et complet des diverses branches de l'art de guerir.* Troisieme division, Chirurgie, Pathologie chirurgicale. Paris, 1839:184-207.

4. Towsend WM. Pterygium. In: Kaufman HE, Barron BA, McDonald MB, Waltam SR eds. *The Cornea.* Churcill Livingstone, 1988:461-83.

5. Terrien F. Operation du Ptérygion. In: Terrien F. *Chirurgie de l'oeil et de ses annexes.* 1921:376-83.

6. Kamel S. Pterygium. Its nature and a new line of treatment. *Br J Ophthalmol* 1946;30:549-63.

7. Stein HA, Slatt BJ, Cook P. Manual of ophthalmic terminology. The C.V. Mosby Company St. Louis Toronto London, 1982:30.

8. Rich L F. Pterygium and pseudopterygium. In: Fraunfelder FT, Roy FH. *Current ocular therapy* 4th ed. Saunders, 1995:474-6.

9. Offret G, Dhermy P, Brini A, Bec P. Anatomie pathologique de l'oeil et de ses annexes. Masson et C.ie, 1971:583.

10. Duke-Helder S. Pterygium. In: Duke-Helder. *Diseases of the outer eye. Conjunctiva.* In: *System of ophthalmology,* vol 8; pt.1, St. Louis, C.V Mosby, 1965:573-85.

11. Moran DJ, Hollows FC. Pterygium and ultraviolet radiation: a positive correlation. *Br J Ophthalmol* 1984;68:343.

12. Taylor HR. Studies on the tear film in climatic drop-let keratopathy and pterygium. *Arch Ophthalmol* vol 98, Jan 1980.

13. Taylor HR et al. Corneal changes associated with chronic UV radiation. *Arch Ophthalmol* 1989; 107:1481.

14. Wittemberg S. Solar radiation and the eye: a review of knowledge relevant to eye care. *Am J Optom Physiol Opt* 1986 Aug;63(8):676-89.

15. Taylor HR, West S, Munoz B, Rosenthal FS, Bressel NM. The long term effects of visible light on the eye. *Arch Ophthalmol* 1993 Mar;111(3):297-8.

16. Roh S, Weiter JJ. Light damage to the eye. *J Fla Med Assoc* 1994 Apr;81(4):248-51.

17. Hect Fondazione, Shoptaugh MG. Winglets of the eye: dominant transmission of early adult pterygium of the conjunctiva. *J Med Genet* 1990 Jun; 27(6):392-4.

18. MacKenzie FD, Hirst LW, Battistutta D, Green A. Risk analysis in the development of pterygia. *Ophthalmology* 1992 Jul;99(7):1056-61.

19. Avisar R. Tear secretion in pterygium. *Harefuah* 1976;92:400-402.

20. Raijv S, Mithal S, Sood AK. Pterygium and dry eye, a clinical correlation. *Indian J Ophthalmol* 1991 Jan-Mar;39(1):15-6.

21. Young RW. The family of sunlight-related eye diseases. *Optom Vis Sci* 1994 Feb;71(2):125-44.

22. Taylor HR. The aetiology of climatic drop-let keratophaty and pterygium. *Br J Ophthalmol* 1980, 64:154-63.

23. Varinli S, Varinli I, Koksal-Erkisi M, Doran Fondazione. Papova virus in patients with pterygium. *Afr J Med* 1994 Jan;40(19):24-6.

24. Liu L, Yang D. Immunological studies on the pathogenesis of pterygium. *Chin Med Sci J* 1993 Jun;8(2):84-8.

25. Klintworth GK. Chronic actinic keratopathy: a condition associated with conjunctival elastosis (pinguecolae) and typified by characteristic extracellular concretion. *Am J Pathol* 1972;67:372.

26. Rodrigues MM, Laibson G, Weimeb S. Corneal elastosis: appearance of band-like keratopathy and spheroidal degeneration. *Arch Ophthalmol* 1975;93:11.

27. Balestrazzi E. Anatomia ed istologia patologica oculare. *Ed Mediche scientifiche Internazionali.* Roma 1994;70-84.

28. Coroneo MT, Muller-Stolzenburg NW, Ho A. Peripheral light focusing by the anterior eye and the ophthalmohelioses. *Ophthalmic Surg* 1991 Dec;22(12):705-11.

29. Mallof Aj, Ho A, Coroneo MT. Influence of corneal shape on limbar light focusing. *Invest Ophthalmol Vis Sci* 1994 Apr;35(5):2592-8.

30. Kwok LS, Coroneo MT. A model for pterygium formation. *Cornea* 1994 May;13(3):219-24.

31. Takazawa S, Ito S, Mita T, Nizuma T, Myyanaga Y, Ishii Y. Inhibitory effect of transilast and active vitamine D3 on proliferation of pterygium tissue. ARVO Annual meeting Fort Lauderdale, Florida May 10-15, 1998.

32. Dushku N, Reid TW. Immunohistochemical evidence that human pterygia originate from an invasion of vimentin-expressing altered limbal epithelial basal cells. *Curr Eye Res* 1994;13,473-81.

33. Pinkerton OD, Hokama Y, Shigemura LA. Immunologic basis for the pathogenesis of pterygium. *Am J Ophthalmol* 1984;98:225-8.

34. Joachim-Velogianni E, Tsironi E, Agnantis N, Datseris G, Psilas K. HLA-DR antigen expression in pterygium epithelial cells and lynphocyte subpopulations: an immonuhistochemistry study. *Ger J Ophthalmol* 1994; 4:123-9.

35. Sivakumar M, Liu Y.P., Tan D.T.H. Singapore National Eye Centre, Singapore. Impression cytology in pterygium. ARVO Annual meeting Fort Lauderdale, Florida May 10-15, 1998.

36. Kaneko M, Takaku I, Katsura N.: Glycosaminoglycans in pterygium tissue and normal conjunctiva. *Jpn J Ophthalmol* 1986;30(2):165-73.

37. Guerzider C, Creuzot-Garcher C, Assem M, Delannoy P, Bron A.M, Bara J. Department of Ophthalmology University of Burgundy, Djion. Laboratory of molecular Genetics, University of Science of Lille, U 55 INSERM, Saint Antoine Hospital, Paris, France. ARVO Annual meeting Fort Lauderdale, Florida May 10-15, 1998.

38. Chen JK, Tsai RJ, Lin SS. Fibroblasts isolated from human pterygia exhibit transformed cell characteristics, *In vitro cell dev biol anim.* 1994 Apr; 30A(4): 243-8.

39. Hilgers J M.: Ptérygion its incidence, heredity and aetiology. *Am J Ophthalmol* 1960;50:635-44.

40. Butrus SI, Farooq Ashraf M, Laby DM, Rabinowitz AL, Tabbara SO, Hidayat Ahamed A. Increased numbers of mastcells in pterygia. *Am J Ophthalmol* 1995;119:236-7.

41. Rohrbach IM, Starc S, Knorr A. Predicting recurent pterygium base on morphologic and immunohistologic parametres. *Ophthalmologie* 1995;92:463-72.

42. Lin BS, Reiter MS, Dreher AW, Fruncht-Pery J, Feldman ST. The effects of pterygia on contrast sensitivity and glare disability. *Am J Ophthalmol* 107:407-410.

43. Giusburg AP, Cannon MW. Comparison of three methods for rapid determination of thresold contrast sensitivity. *Invest Ophthalmol Vis Sci* 1983;24:788.

44. Hirsch RP, Nadler MP, Miller D. Clinical performance of a disability glare tester. *Arch Ophthalmol* 1984; 102:1633.

45. Hochbaum DR, Moskovitz SF, Wirtschaffer JD. A quantitative analysis of astigmatism induced by pterygium. *Journal of Biomechanics* 1977;10:735-746.

46. Oldenburg JB, Garbus J, McDonnell JM, McDonnell PJ. Conjunctival pterygia. Mechanism of corneal topographic changes. *Cornea.* 1990 Jul; 9(3):200-4.

47. Amsler M. Pterygium causing corneal astigmatism. *Ophthalmologica* 1953;126:52-54.

48. Bedrossian RH. The effects of pterygium surgery on refraction and corneal curvature.

49. Hansen A. Astigmatism and surface phenomena in pterygium. *Acta Ophthalmologica* (Copenaghen) 1980; 58(29):174-181.

50. Perdriel M.G. Traitment du pterygion par injiections sous-conjonctivales d'hydrocortisone. *Bull Soc Ophtalmol* Fr 1958;675-8.

51. Ellis OP. Terapia e farmacologia oculare. *Medical Book*s. Palermo 1986.

52. Frucht-Pery J, Siganos C.S, Solomon A, Shvartzenberg T, Richards C, Trinquand C. Department of Ophthalmology, Hadassah University Hospital Jerusalem, Israel; Laboratoire Chauvin, Montpellier, France. ARVO Annual meeting Fort Lauderdale, Florida May 10-15, 1998.

53. Proto F, Malagola R, Carnevale C. Effetto dello Yag laser e dell'argon laser sulla vascolarizzazione dello pterigio. *Boll Ocul* 1988;67:395-9.

54. Saiffudin S, Baum KL. Reccurent pterygia-laser therapy: a preliminary report. *Indian J Ophthalmol* 1993 Apr;41(1):17-9.

55. Cornand G. Pterygium. Clinical course and treatment. *Rev Int Trach Pathol Ocul Tro Subtop Sante Publique* 1989;66(3-4):31-108.

56. Bende T, Seiler T, Wollensak J. Superficial ablation of the cornea using the excimer laser (193 nm). *Fortschr-Ophthalmol* 1989;86(6):589-91.

57. Seiler T, Schnelle B, Wollensak J. Pterygium excision using 193-nm excimer laser smoothing and topical mytomicin C. *Ger J Ophthalmol* 1992; 1(6):429-31.

58. Krag S, Ehlers N. Excimer laser treatment of pterygium. *Acta Ophthalmologica* 1992 Aug; 70(4):530-3.

59. Walter AJ. Another look al pterygium surgery with postoperative beta radiation. *Ophthalmic Plast Surg* 1994;10:247-52.

60. De Keizer RJ, Asart van der Berg M, Baartse WJ. Results of pterygium excision with Sr90 irradiation, lamellar keratoplasty and conjunctival flap. *Doc Ophtgalmology* 1987;6,33-44.

61. Wesberry Jm, Wesberry JM Sr. Optimal use of beta irradiation in the treatment of pterygia. *South Med J* 1993 Jun;86(6):633-7.

62. Neal AJ, Irwin C, Hope-Stone HF. The role of stronzium 90 beta irradiation in the management of pterygium. *Clin Onc R Coll Rad* 1991 Mar;3(2):105-9.

63. Wilder RB, Buatti JM, Kittelson JM, Shimm DS, Harari PM, Rogoff EE, et al. Pterygium treated with excision and postoperative beta irradiation. *Int Radiation Oncology Biol Phys* 1992;23:533-7.

64. Campbell OR, Amendola BE, Brady LW.: Recurrent pterygia: results of postoperative treatment with Sr-90 applicators. *Radiology* 1990;174:565-6.

65. Beyer DC. Pterygia: single fraction postoperative beta irradiation. *Radiology* 1991 Feb;178(2):569-71.

66. Aswad MI, Baum J. Optimal time for post-operative irradiation of pterygia. *Ophthalmology* 1987; 94:1450-1.

67. Paryani SB, Scott WP, Wells JW, Johnson DW, Chobe RJ, Kuruvilla A, et al, and North Florida Pterygium Study Group. Management of pterygium with surgery and radiation therapy. *Int J Radiation Oncology Biol Phys* 1993;28:101-3.

68. Bahrassa F, Datta R. Postoperative beta radiation treatment of pterygium. *Int J Radiation Oncology Biol Phys* 1983;9:679-84.

69. Chayakul V. Postoperative Mytomicin C eye-drop and beta-radiation in the treatment of pterygia. *J Med Assoc Thai* 1991 Sept;774(9):373-6.

70. MacKenzie FD, Hirst LW, Kynaston B, Bain C. Recurrence rate and complications after beta therapy for pterygia. *Ophthalmology* 1991 Dec; 98(12):1176-80; discussion 178.

71. Dusenbery KE, Alul IH, Holland EJ, Khan FM, Levitt SH. Beta irradiation of recurrent pterygia: results and complications. *Int J Radiat Oncol Biol Phys* 1992; 24(2):315-20.

72. Moriarty AP, Crawford GJ, Mac Allister IL, Constabile IJ. Severe corneosclera infection. A complication of beta irradiation cleral necrosis following pterygium excission. Comment in *Arch Ophthalmol* 1994 Aug; 112(8):1016-77.

73. Tarr KH, Constable IJ. Late complications of pterygium treatment. *Br J Ophtalmol* 1980;64:496-505.

74. Eong KG, Tseng PS, Lim AS. Scleral necrosis and infection 15 years following pterygium excision. *Singapore Med J* 1995 Apr;36(2):232-4.

75. Moriarty AP, Crawford GJ, Mac Allister IL, Constabile IJ. Fungal corneoscleritis complicating beta-irradiation-induced scleral necrosis following pterygium excision. *Eye* 1993;7(pt4):525-8.

76. Farrell PL, Smith RE. Bacterial corneoscleritis complicating pterygium excision. *Am J Ophthalmol* 1989 May;107(5):515-7.

77. Robert Y, Pauli L, Gysin P, Gloor B, Hendrickson P. Protracted ruthenium treatment of recurrent pterygium. *Graefes Arch Clin Exp Ophthalmol.* 1992; 230 (3):233-6.

78. Nakamura M, Yamamoto M. DNA interstrand crosslinking agents and human ocular fibroblasts: differenzial sensitivity to mytomicin C and cisdiamodichloroplatinum. *Exp Eye Res* 1994;59:53-62.

79. Frucht-Pery J, Charalambos S, Ilsar M. Intraoperative application of topical Mytomicin C for pterygium surgery. *Ophthalmology* 1996;103:674-7.

80. Frucht-Pery J, Ilsar M, Hemo I. Single dosage of mytomicin C for prevention of recurrent pterygium: preliminary report. *Cornea* 1994;13:411-3.

81. Heiligenhaus A, Akova Y, Lung E, Schrenk M, Waubke TN. Pterygium excision with intraoperative administration of low-dosage mytomicin C. *Ophthalmologe* 1995;92:458-62.

82. Cano-Parra J, Diaz-Llopis M, Maldonado MJ, Menezo JL. Prospective trial of intraoperative mytomicin C in the treatment of primary pterygium. *Br J Ophthalmol* 1995;79:439-41.

83. Mastropasqua L, Carpineto P, Ciancagini M, Lobefalo L, Gallenga PE. Effectiveness of intraoperative mytomicin C in the treatment of recurrente pterygium. *Ophthalmologica* 1994;208:247-9.

84. Magdi Helal, Nabil Messiha, Ashraf Amayem, Akef El-Maghraby, Zakaria Elsherif, Mostafa Dabees. Intraoperative mytomicin-C versus postoperative topical mytomicin-C drops for the treatment of pterygium. *Ophthalmic Surg Lasers* 1996;27:674-8.

85. Singh G, Wilson MR, Foster CS. Mitomycin eye drops as treatment for pterygium. *Ophthalmology* 1988; 95:813-21

86. Rachmiel R, Leiba H, Levartovsky S. Results of treatment with topical mitomycin C 0.02% following excision of primary pterygium. *Br J Ophthalmol* 1993; 77:433-5.

87. Mahar PS, Nwokora GE. Role of mitomycin C in pterygium surgery. *Br J Ophthalmol* 1993;77:433-5.

88. Rosenthal G, Shoham A Lifshitz T, Biedner B Yassur Y. The use of mitomycin C in pterygium surgery. *Ann Ophthalmol* 1993;25:427-8.

89. Ewing-Chow DA, Romanchuk KG, Gilmour GR, Underhill JH, Clirmenhaga DB. Corneal melting after pterygium removal followed by topical mitomycin C therapy. *Can J Ophthalmol* 1992;27:197-9.

90. Rubinfield RS, Pfister RR, Stein RM, Foster CS, Martin NF, Stoleru S et al. Serious complications of topical mitomycin C after pterygium surgery. *Ophthalmology* 1992;99:1647-54.

91. Marder WE, Ogawa GSH., Schluter ML. University of New Mexico Health Sciences Center, Albuqueque, NM. Late scleral necrosis after pterygium surgery with mitomycin C. ARVO Annual meeting Fort Lauderdale, Florida May 10-15, 1998.

92. Frucht-Pery J, Ilsar M. The use of low-dosage Mitomy-

cin C for prevention of recurrent pterygium. *Ophthalmology* 1994;101:759-62.

93. Hayasaka S, Noda S, Yamamoto Y, Setogawa T. Postoperative instillation of low-dose mitomycin C in the treatment of prymary pterygium. *Am J Ophthalmol* 1988;106:715-8.

94. Chen PP, Ariyasu RG, Venu Kaza, Labree LD, McDonnell PJ. A randomized trial comparing mitomycin C and conjunctival autograft after excision of primary pterygium. *Am J Ophthalmol* 1995; 120:151-60.

95. Hara T, Shoji E, Hara T, Obara Y. Pterygium surgery using the principle of contact inhibition and a limbal transplanted pedicle conjunctival strip. *Ophthalmic Surg* 1994;25:95-8.

96. Lee J.R, Lee J.S, Oum B.S, Kim Y.S. Department of Ophthalmology, College of Medicine, Central Research Laboratory, Pusan National University, Pusan Korea. A evaluation of efficacy of Mytomicin-C (0.002%-0.04%) in metabolic activity and cytotoxicity in pterygium. ARVO Annual meeting Fort Lauderdale, Florida May 10-15, 1998.

97. Troutman RC. Microsurgery of the anterior segment of the eye. Vol 1. *Introduction and basic techniques.* Mosby Company 1974:203-258.

98. Heilman K, Paton D. Cornea Glaucoma Lens Vol.II di Atlas of ophthalmic surgery-techniques-complications. Thieme Verlag Stuttgardt-New York Thieme *Medical Publishers Inc.* New York 1987;1.34-1.39.

99. De Rotth A. Plastic repair of conjunctival defects with fetal membrane. *Arch Ophthalmol* 1940; 23:522-5.

100. Lavary W. Lime burns of conjunctiva and cornea treated with amnioplastin graft. *Trans Ophthalmol Soc UK* 1946;66:668-71.

101. Trelford JD, Trelford-Sauder M. The amnion in surgery, past and present. *Am J Obset Gynecol* 1979;134:833-45.

102. Colocho G, Graham WP, Greene AE, Matheson DW, Lynch D. Human amniotic membrane as a physiologic wound dressing. *Arch Surg* 1974;109:370-3.

103. Prasad JK, Feller I, Thompson PD. Use of amnion for the treatment of Stevens-Johnsons syndrome. *J Trauma* 1986;26:945-6.

104. Zohar Y, Talmi YP, Fincklstein Y, et al. Use of human amniotic membrane in otolaryngologic practice. *Laryngoscope* 1987;97:978-80.

105. Shimazaki J, Shinozaki N, Tsubota K. Transplantation of amniotic membrane and limbal autograft for patients with recurrent pterygium associated with symblefaron. *Br J Ophthalmol* 1998;82:235-240.

106. Thoft RA. Keratoepithelioplasty. *Am J Ophthalmol* 1984;97:1-6.

107. Pearlman G, Susal AL, Hushaw J, Bartlett RE. Recurrent pterygium and treatment with lamellar keratoplasty with presentation of a technique to limit recurrence: a preliminary report. *Ann Ophthalmol* 1970;2:763-71.

108. Vrabec MP, Weisenthal RW, Elsing SH. Subconjunctival fibrosis after conjunctival autograft. *Cornea* 1993;12:181-3.

109. Prabhasawat P, Barton K, Burkett G, Scheffer CG, Tseng CG. Comparison of conjunctival autografts, amniotic membrane grafts, and primary closure for pterygium excision. *Ophthalmology* 1997;104(6): 974-85.

110. DoWlut MS, Laflamme MY. Les pterygions recidivants: frequence et correction par autogreffe conjonctivale. *Can J Ophthalmol* 1981;16:119-20.

111. Cornand G. Le pterygion in: Terrien F. *Chirurgie de l'oeil et des annexes.* 1921:376-83.

112. Arffa R C. Pterygium. In: Arffa RC. Grayson's Diseases of the Cornea. *Mosby Year Book*, 1991:342-5.

113. Flament U, Speeg-Schatz CI,Weber M.: Etat actuel du traitement du ptérygion. *J Fr Ophtalmol* 1993;16: 401-10.

114. Hampton Roy F. Ocular syndromes and systemic diseases. 2nd ed. W.B. Saunders Company 1989:361.

115. Klintworth GK. Degenerations, Depositions and miscellaneous reactions of the ocular anterior segment. In: Pathobiology of ocular diseases - a dynamic approach. 2nd ed. Garner A, Klintworth GK, 1996: 743-52.

116. Kanski JJ. Clinical ophthalmology - a systematic approach. 2nd ed. Butterworths, 1989:79.

117. Boudet C, Millet P. Ptérygion. In: *Encyclopedie Med Chir.*, Paris, *Ophthalmologie* 1983.

118. Barraquer J, Rutlan J. Surgery of the anterior segment of the eye. Surgery of the cornea Vol. 2 - *Keratectomies, conjunctivoplasties, lamellar keratoplasty, penetrating keratoplasty.* Barcelona 1971:123-30.

119. Jaros PA, DeLuise VP. Pinguaeculae and pterygia. *Surv Ophthalmol* 1988;33:41-49.

120. Boyd BF. Highlights of Ophthalmology World Atlas series of ophthalmic surgery volume 1. 1993:30-40.

121. Wong Wayne W. Behavior of skin grafts in treatment of recurrent pterygium. *Ann Ophthalmol* 1977;9:352-6.

122. Bianchi C, Bandello F, Brancato R. Manuale di oftalmologia essenziale. Ghedini editore Milano, 1995: 200-2.

123. Hirst LW, Sebban A, Chant D. Pterygium recurrence time. *Ophthalmology* 1994;101:755-8.

124. Isler MS, Delmar R, Caldwell R. Peripheral diseases (Terrien's diseases and recurrent pterygium). In: Brightbill FS ed. *Corneal surgery-theory, technique, and tissue.* The C.V. Mosby Company, 1986;387-95.

125. Camellin M, Capobianco W, Merlin U. Laser ad eccimeri: applicazioni in chirurgia non refrattiva. *Contattologia medica e chirurgia refrattiva* 1990;2: 163-171.

PART B

Contributors

RAFAEL I. BARRAQUER, M.D.

DONALD T.H. TAN, M.D.

ABRAHAM SOLOMON, M.D. — SCHEFFER C.G. TSENG, M.D., Ph.D

JOSEPH FRUCHT-PERY, M.D. — CHARALAMBOS S. SIGANOS, M.D.

ROBERT L. PHILLIPS, M.D.

1

PERSONAL APPROACH TO PTERYGIUM

Rafael I. Barraquer, M.D.

INTRODUCTION

Successful management of a pterygium requires a clear understanding of its pathogenesis and the recognition of the clinical features that indicate risk of recurrence. In spite of being one of the oldest known ocular conditions – at least since Susruta, over 3000 years ago[1], and the subject of one of the ophthalmic surgical procedures most frequently performed throughout the world, it still poses a disturbing therapeutic challenge.

The difficulty starts from the very definition of the lesion. The usual approach is descriptive, as in a dictionary entry: *Pterygium: an abnormal mass of tissue arising from the conjunctiva of the inner corner of the eye that obstructs vision by growing over the cornea.*[2] Conceptually, this is not a great improvement over the popular idea behind the various colloquial definitions – in Spain it is commonly called *palmera* (palm tree) or *uña* (nail), or the Greek word for "small wing" from which the medical term derives.

We still hesitate when attempting a classification and usually group a pterygium among the "conjunctival degenerations". This reflects our uncertainties about its nature and pathogenesis, resorting to a process of exclusion: pterygia are not neoplastic, nor caused by trauma, infection or inflammation. Whenever a lesion resembling a pterygium is clearly secondary to any of these etiologic factors, it is called a "pseudopterygium". What then is a genuine pterygium? What causes it?

Before presenting my current techniques for the treatment of a pterygium, a review of the clinical and pathological facts may help in understanding the pathogenesis and in predicting its natural behavior and response to surgery.

CLINICAL FEATURES

The above cited dictionary definition of a pterygium can be extended and refined by commenting on the individual features:

1) *"An abnormal mass of tissue...":* Three portions can be distinguished in this triangular, band-shaped lesion: a "head" or apex preceded by a "glass cap" or halo (avascular zone), and a fibrovascular "body". These structures differentiate pterygia from pingueculae, pseudopterygia and other limbal lesions. Additional general morphological features include:

a) *Band-shaped.* This grossly distinguishes pterygia from the more prevalent pingueculae. These can be whitish, flat and atrophic (Stage I), or raised, mound-like and vascular (Stage II), but as a rule small and rounded, and do not show tendency to invade the cornea.

b) *Horizontal.* This relates pterygia to the interpalpebral fissure, suggesting an external, environmental etiologic factor. Pseudopterygia, on the contrary, may develop in any quadrant.

c) *Triangular.* The classical shape suggests an oriented process, as the pterygium head grows over the cornea and "drags" the fibrovascular body. In contradistinction, limbal tumors tend to spread in all directions or around the limbus.

d) *Bilateral.* Most cases show some involvement of both eyes, although asymmetric– which explains that only a third may be counted as properly bilateral.[3]

2) *"...arising from the conjunctiva..."*: The fleshy appearance of the pterygium differentiates it both from the normal surrounding conjunctiva and from the usually duller neoplasia or dysplasia. However, the latter can rarely develop over a pterygium. The degree of fleshiness (vs. translucency) has been shown to be a risk factor for recurrence after surgery.[4] Additional features include:

a) *Vascularity.* Redness is the common reason for the patient's cosmetic concern, but congestion also indicates activity and a tendency to grow. The typically radial orientation of the vessels indicates its head pulls the pterygium body.

b) *Adherence.* While the head adheres firmly to the cornea, the body is not attached to the sclera. However, an instrument cannot be passed under it, as may be the case with a pseudopterygium.

3) *"...of the inner corner of the eye..."*: Pterygia are typically nasal. Although some 10% of cases may present with a second, temporal lesion, these are extremely rare as an isolated occurrence.[5]

4) *"...that obstructs vision..."*: As a pterygium invades the optical area of the cornea, decreased visual acuity and contrast sensitivity, and increased glare will ensue. However, similar disturbances can be caused earlier by high regular or irregular astigmatism induced at a distance.

This may be the result of distortion of the cornea by tractional forces or disruption of the tear film itself.[6] A very taut pterygium can even cause diplopia.

5) *"...growing over the cornea"*: Pterygia tend to advance over the cornea but almost never pass the corneal apex. The actual course of the growth varies widely. The patient frequently describes a rapid initial development along a few months, but the previous presence of a pinguecula-like lesion for a longer time is commonly admitted. Then the advancement slows and may cease (and may even regress to a flat scar), or show episodes of reactivation, encroaching progressively on the cornea. Additional features include:

a) *Symptoms.* The intermittent periods of growth are associated to irritation, burning, foreign body sensation, photophobia and tearing, either caused by the tear film disruption or by the concurrent inflammation.

b) *Staining.* Many pterygia show punctate staining with either fluorescein or rose bengal and sometimes over the adjacent cornea, even with dellen. This is a sign of tear film disturbance, which is the basis base for one pathogenetic theory and a possible clue to aggressivity.

c) *Stocker's line.* A brownish iron line in the corneal epithelium may appear bordering the head, indicating tear pooling. Although this could happen with any elevated lesion at this site, it suggests chronicity and a slow growth.[7]

d) *Ilots of Fuchs.* As the pterygium evolves, the apex develops the cap, which may show satellite opacities projecting towards the center of the cornea. These are an additional hint of growth tendency.

HISTOPATHOLOGY

The classic pathologic feature of both pterygia and pingueculae – but not of recurrent pterygia – is elastotic degeneration of the subepithelial substantia propria. However, this abnormal connective tissue is not digested by elastase, which only acts on normal elastin.[8] The characteristic staining would be the result of degenerated maturational forms of elastic fibers produced by abnormal fibroblastic activity.[9] In fact, increased number of fibroblasts is a common finding. These changes are similar to actinic degeneration of the skin, in which ultraviolet (UV) radiation stimulates fibroblasts to secrete elastic precursors.

The hypertrophic and degenerated collagenous tissue which constitutes the bulk of the pterygium mass is populated by dilated vessels both original (conjunctival, Tenon's, and episcleral) and of new formation, which suggests increased angiogenesis. The overlying epithelium may show variable thickness but appear otherwise normal. Abnormalities in the mucus glycoprotein secretion[10] may contribute to tear film dysfunction. Some cases show changes such as acanthosis, dyskeratosis, and even squamous cell metaplasia, constituting pterygium with dysplasia.

The fibrovascular tissue at the apex invades the cornea between Bowman's layer and the epithelial basement membrane. An advancing row of fibroblasts appears in the region of the cap, eventually digesting and focally interrupting Bowman's layer. This allows the invading tissue to penetrate the corneal stroma, which explains the head's firm anchoring[11]. The immediately overlying epithelial cells have been identified immunohistochemically as altered limbal basal epithelial stem cells (AE1 positive and AE5 negative)[12] that have become migratory, as suggested by their expression of vimentin.[13] These "pterygium cells" also express an abnormal amount of the p53 protein,[14] a fact that has important pathogenetic implications.

PATHOGENESIS

The causes and mechanisms of pterygium development have been the subject of many theories. Recent basic findings are shifting the focus from the conjunctiva to the limbal basal epithelial stem cells as the site of the primary dysfunction.

Solar irradiation

Most evidence appears to support that solar ex-posure,[15] and especially UV-B radiation, is the main etiologic factor. The epidemiological data clearly show a relationship between pterygia and warm climates, especially if dry and windy (i.e., less cloudy), with a strong correlation with the lower latitudes.[16,17] The lack of solar protection such as spectacles (or even a hat) was found to be statistically significant.[18]

A recent study strongly relates pterygium and sun exposure with a dose-response curve and, contrary to previous reports, irrespective of the period of life involved.[19] Above the 40° parallel, pterygia are rare and mostly confined to outdoor workers such as farmers and fishermen.[20] The occupational factor probably explains the male predominance in some studies, which is not found when considering only indoor workers.[21] Obviously, working indoors does not preclude a high solar exposure in the tropics, at least during part of the life. Also supporting an UV-B etiology, older studies associating pterygia pterygium with welding have been replaced with a rare prevalence when adequate UV-protection is used.[22]

Irritative, Inflammatory and Local Drying Theories

An earlier group of irritative or inflammatory theories, dating at least from Scarpa,[23] could explain the increased incidence found among some indoor workers exposed to dust.[24] A type I hypersensitivity reaction to dust or pollen has been supported by the finding of IgG and IgE.[25]

Whatever the initial cause, most pterygia appear to develop from a preexisting pinguecula. Once a local elevation is produced next to the limbus, the disturbance of the tear film resulting in dryness of the adjacent cornea could trigger the progressive fibrovascular invasion as a cicatricial response. This mechanism was first proposed by José I. Barraquer[26] and supported by others. However, corneal micro-ulcerations and dellen are only rarely seen in active pterygia.

Mechanism of the Nasal Localization

The horizontal, interpalpebral location of pterygia is explained by the environmental etiology.

Why then the nasal predominance? Miller hypothesized some irritant factor present in the sweat, and demonstrated using rose bengal that the sweat flowing down from the forehead enters the nasal conjunctiva through the inner canthus.[27]

If UV light is the causing factor, why pterygia are rare on the more-exposed, temporal side? Arenas was the first to sustain that the light entering the temporal side would by focused on the nasal perilimbal sector.[28] A mathematical model has concluded that the cornea can concentrate the albedo UV radiation by a factor of 20 on the nasal side of the limbus.[29]

Limbal Stem Cell Dysfunction Theory

Most pathologically based theories focused on the prominent elastotic and collagenous degenerative changes, and supported a fibroblast damage by UV radiation as the main process, similar to the skin model of solar damage. However, recent work by Dushku et al.[12–14] suggest a primarily limbal epithelial stem cell dysfunction, with loss of the junctional barrier that separates the conjunctival and corneal epithelia and a centripetal migration of mutant limbal basal cells (pterygium cells).

Pterygium would actually be "a migrating limbus", the conjunctival fibrovascular tissue being only secondarily attracted.

An abnormal production of the p53 protein in the basal limbal epithelial stem cells, found in stage II pingueculae (elevated, vascularized), pterygia, and limbal tumors, but not in fibroblasts, suggests a common pathogenesis for all these lesions.[14]

The p53 protein is the product of a tumor-suppressor gene, which has been called "the guardian of the genome" and a common target of various carcinogenic factors. In normal cells, when the DNA is damaged (as by UV radiation), the p53 protein arrests the nuclear activity allowing for extra repair time before the S phase. If the repair fails, p53 may trigger cell death by apoptosis.[30] However, if the p53 gene itself is damaged, this programmed cell-death mechanism is impaired allowing for further mutations in other genes, in spite of an increased amount of abnormal p53 protein.

In the limbus, this would lead to a multistep progression from pingueculae to pterygia and occasionally to limbal neoplasia *(Figure 1-1).*[14]

UV-B exposure is probably the main mutagenic factor while the human papilloma virus, although incidentally found in some cases, has been ruled out as a cofactor.[31] The critical step would be the transformation of the normally static, limbal epithelial basal stem cells into altered, migratory cells, as revealed by the expression of vimentin.[13] These cells also overproduce Transforming Growth Factor Beta (TGF-β), which can explain many of the tissue changes observed in pterygia: (1) A reduced number of epithelial cell layers. (2) Increased angiogenesis. (3) Monocyte and fibroblast accumulation, with both (4) normal collagen deposition and (5) collagenase activation causing Bowman's dissolution. (6) Anterior fibroblast migration to form the ilots of Fuchs, and (7) increased motility of the pterygium cells by collagenase-induced dissolution of the epithelial hemidesmosomes. Although the UV effect on the fibroblasts can explain the initial elastotic degeneration, they would not be pathogenic for pterygia.[31]

The main therapeutic consequence of this theory is the emphasis on the restoration of the normal limbal barrier. It is not an aggressive conjunctival tissue "pushing" into the cornea, but rather being "dragged" by the migrating altered limbal cells of the apex. The pterygium cells initially infiltrate the conjunctival and corneal epithelium surrounding he originating pinguecula in a centrifugal manner, before initiating their directional migration towards the corneal apex. Together with a documented superficial spread of these normally indistinguishable cells, this could explain recurrences in spite of large excisions and mucous membrane grafts, calling for the use of antimetabolites or physical therapy to eradicate them.

While recurrent pterygia do not show elastotic degeneration but keloid-like fibrous tissue hypertrophy, they do have p53-positive cells, indicating that any significant number of pterygium cells remaining in the corneal epithelium after surgery could induce a recurrence by secondarily attracting new fibrovascular tissue.

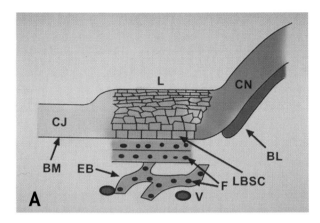
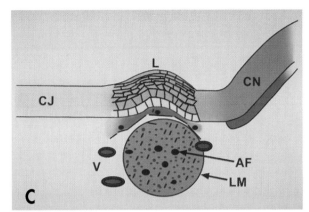
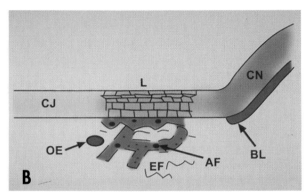
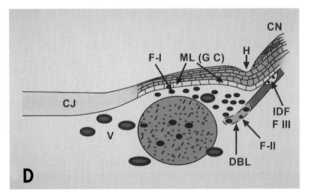

Figure 1-1. *Limbal stem cell dysfunction pathogenesis of pterygium.* **A.** *Normal limbus (CJ = conjunctiva; L = limbus; CN = cornea; BM = basement membrane; LBSC = limbal basal stem cells; BL = Bowman's layer; EB = eosinophilic bundles; F = fibroblasts; V = blood vessel).* **B.** *Stage I pinguecula: atrophic changes predominate with decreased epithelial cell layers (L) and fibroblasts (AF), obliterative endarteritis (OE) causing avascular scars, irregular fragmenting of bundles, which become thin and basophilic, and formation of elastotic fibers (EF).* **C.** *Stage II pinguecula: p53 mutation appears in LBSC and there is increase in altered fibroblasts (AF), angiogenesis and elastogenesis causing a microfibrillar lobule (LM).* **D.** *Pterygium: additional mutations induce migratory behavior in the p53 mutated LBSC, becoming a migrating limbus (ML) which grows over the corneal BM, followed by conjunctival epithelium and stroma. There is increased angiogenesis and the underlying fibroblasts produce altered elastic material (F-I). Those at the apex (F-II) produce collagenase and dissolve the Bowman's layer (DBL) and may migrate over it forming the ilots of Fuchs (IDS). There is a decrease in epithelial cell layers. GC = glass cap; H = halo. An alternative pathway from pinguecula state II may lead to limbal tumor if the additional mutations induce oncogene activation in non-migratory LBSC (not shown). From Dushku & Reid,*[14] *with permission.*

TREATMENT

Most textbooks and reviews dedicate a few paragraphs to prevention and medical treatment, including sunglasses and avoidance of irritating environments, ocular lubricants, vasoconstrictors and anti-inflammatory drops, either non-steroidal (NSAI) or mild steroids with the usual concerns. While this can be helpful in mild cases, many patients will end up requiring or asking for surgery. Before presenting my personal current approach I will briefly comment on the available surgical alternatives and adjunctive therapies, under the light of the current pathogenetic theories.

Surgical Alternatives

The variety of therapies proposed for the treatment of pterygia implies that we are far from knowing the ideal method. The abundance of the related literature precludes an attempt to analyze it here in depth, and excellent reviews can be found in several papers,[1,5,32,33] textbooks, and elsewhere in this book. However, a number of reasons hinder the validity and usefulness of the information available:

• The success of any surgical technique depends on many factors difficult to standardize, beginning with the surgeon. Sometimes minor variations can be critical, which may not be clearly portrayed in the papers.

- While the usual measure of success is the rate (or absence) of recurrences, we lack a clear definition of what is a recurrence, so these figures are difficult to compare.

- Any analysis of the results should take into account the variable behavior of pterygia and the possible associated conditions (trachoma, etc.). Many series do not consider the (hardly definable) different degrees of aggressivity among primary cases and even mix primary and recurrent cases.

- The different pathogenesis of primary and recurrent pterygia has not always been recognized but is an essential factor to be taken into consideration when analyzing the results of the different modalities.

Avulsion

The very oldest technique[1] and still advocated by some surgeons, based on its simplicity and minimal trauma, which would minimize scarring.[32] However, it may be difficult to unify what each author really considers under this heading.

Simple Excision

The classical *bare sclera* procedure was advocated at least since D'Ombain.[1] Currently its high recurrence rates (1/3 to 2/3, not much better than with avulsion) are used as a baseline to compare newer techniques. This approach is mostly based on two ideas: that recurrences depend on (a) regrowth from "aggressive" conjunctiva, Tenon's, or fibrovascular remnants, and (b) the degree of surface irregularity left.

Addressing the first, the resection is meticulous and the conjunctival borders are fixated away from the limbus to allow for the corneal epithelium to cover the bare sclera, preventing fibrovascular regrowth.[34]

The goal of "reaching normal conjunctiva" is limited by the increased scarring as a larger area of sclera remains exposed and the corneal epithelium fails to cover it before a granulation tissue devel-

ops. The second idea originates the various techniques of keratectomy, scraping, burring and cleaning of the head's bed to obtain a smooth surface. But even the use of the most sophisticated instrument, an excimer laser, may result in a fiasco (91% recurrence).[35]

According to the limbal stem cell pathogenetic theory, a decreased recurrence after any of such limbal resections would depend on the *extensiveness of epithelium removal (not the depth!)*, and thus its success in eradicating all pterygium cells that may invade normal-appearing tissue.[14] This is limited by the fact that a too extensive limbectomy may preclude the corneal epithelium or the normal limbal stem cells from adjacent sectors to restore the limbal barrier,[36] leading to conjuntivalization - actually a "false" recurrence.

Excision With Primary Closure

This group of techniques is based on the ideas of: (a) "bringing healthy conjunctiva" to the dissected area, (b) to create a smooth surface, and (c) a "barrier" preventing the recurring tissue to reach the cornea. Numerous modalities have been developed with varying success, from rotational flaps to sliding flaps to Z-plasties, among others.

The covering of the scleral bed should reduce the scarring response, but even normal conjunctiva can be the source of a recurrence, particularly if the causal pterygium cells still remain at the corneal margin. If this has been scraped or excised, the sliding flaps[37] may actually bring in normal limbal epithelium, but they might also contain pterygium cells if the resection has been small.

Transposition of the Pterygium Head

This idea original of Desmarres[38] also gave place to diverse variants. The underlying conceptions are similar to those of primary closure but simplifying the procedure and minimizing trauma by avoiding the need of excision. Instead, the pterygium head was diverted away from the cornea. Apart from the often-poor cosmetic results, the persistence of the causal cells explains a high recurrence rate.

Conjunctival and Limbal Autografts

The use of free grafts of bulbar conjunctiva, from the same or opposite eye, to cover the excision site dates back to Elschnig,[1] but was revived by José I. Barraquer[39] and by Kenyon et al.[40] The recurrence rate dropped to about 5%, even with recurrent pterygia. Compared to primary closure with flaps, autografts use of a more reliable source of conjunctiva (probably without pterygium cells), avoid closure under tension, and are able to cover larger defects of up to 15 by 15 mm. The disadvantages are a more laborious technique and the possibility of complications at the donor site.

If the tissue is harvested down to the limbus and placed respecting the anatomic orientation, this will actually be a form of limbal transplantation, therefore having more chances of restoring the limbal barrier, provided the pterygium cells have been completely removed from the cornea. A further step of the same idea is the use of a limbal graft "proper",[41] which may be necessary after extensive circumferential damage or excision.

Other Autologous Grafts (mucous membrane, skin)

As alternatives to conjunctiva, a number of autologous tissues have been proposed for a long time, including skin (Gifford), buccal (Svoboda)[1] or nasal[42] mucous membrane. Although their histological nature differs from conjunctiva and do not include limbal stem cells, they may serve well the role of covering the sclera, facilitating surface reconstruction. There is always a question about their cosmetic appearance, especially with skin.

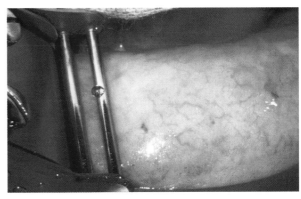

Figure 1-3. *Obtaining a thin buccal mucous membrane graft from the inner lower lip with the Castroviejo electrokeratome. The mucosa is clamped and infiltrated with saline.*

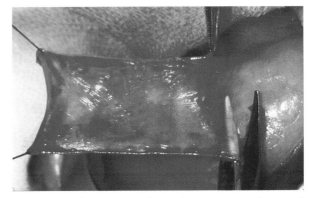

Figure 1-4. *Final scissors cut to obtain a large mucous membrane graft from the lower lip.*

The Castroviejo electrokeratome makes possible the harvesting of thin (0.2 to 0.3 mm and up to 15 by 40 mm), almost transparent pieces of mucous membrane from the inner lower lip *(Figure 1-4 to 1-8)*. Extensive, recurrent cases with multiple heads and associated symblepharon may require grafts of this size that cannot be obtained from the conjunctiva *(Figures 1-5 to 1-8)*.

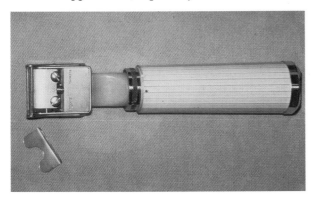

Figure 1-2. *The Castroviejo electrokeratome with the 0.2 mm gauge plate.*

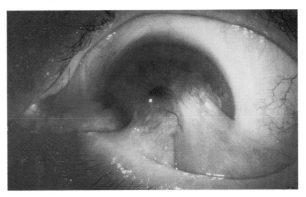

Figure 1-5. *Multiply recurrent pterygium with several heads or pseudopterygia and lower broad symblepharon.*

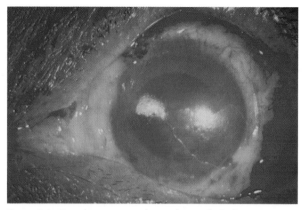

Figure 1-6. *Buccal mucous membrane thin graft. Early postoperative appearance (cornea stained with fluorescein). After the resection of the lesions and superficial keratectomy, there were no deep corneal opacities but the denuded area was too large for a conjunctival autograft. The mucosa is in place, also reforming the inferior fornix. Note the transparent (not pink) appearance of this thin graft.*

Allografts (corneal, limbal, amniotic membrane)

If there is a significant thinning of the cornea or sclera due previous surgeries, the restoration of the eye wall will require a corneal transplant. Tectonic grafts are usually lamellar and may be round or have special shapes (horseshoe, crescent, fusiform, trapezoid, etc.). A penetrating keratoplasty may be necessary to remove full thickness opacities in the visual axis *(Figures 1-9 to 1-12)*. It has been argued that the corneal tissue is a better barrier to pterygium regrowth. This may actually be the result of normal limbal stem cells present and, in fact, a horseshoe keratoplasty or sclerokeratoplasty will probably include a limbal allograft.

The application of amniotic membrane[43] is the last but not least promising approach to resurfacing

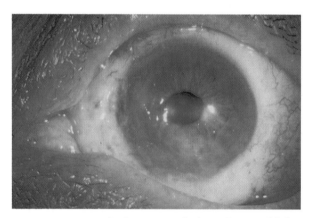

Figure 1-7. *One month after surgery, the lower fornix and bulbar conjunctiva are well reformed but the peripheral cornea in not yet epithelialized, requiring a therapeutic contact lens.*

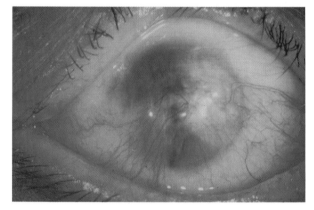

Figure 1-9. *Double headed pterygia or pseudopterygia after multiple failures. There is thinning and deep scarring in the visual axis. (Courtesy of Dr. J. Temprano).*

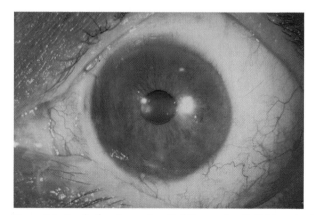

Figure 1-8. *Result after six months with full corneal epithelial integrity and no recurrence of the pterygia.*

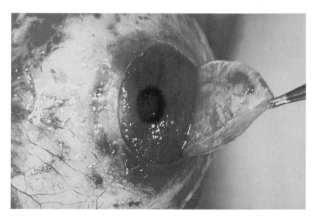

Figure 1-10. *Intraoperative appearance after resection of the pterygia and of the lamellar button. (Courtesy of Dr. J. Temprano).*

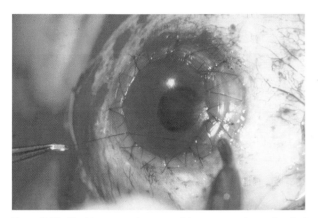

Figure 1-11. *Final intraoperative stage of the reconstructive and optical lamellar keratoplasty. (Courtesy of Dr. J. Temprano).*

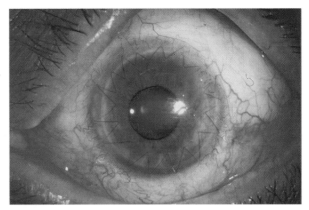

Figure 1-12. *Result after two months with restoration of the corneal transparency and no recurrences. (Courtesy of Dr. J. Temprano).*

after a pterygium excision. It is actually a form of allograft with low antigenicity and multiple features favorable for ocular surface reconstruction, including its availability in large pieces.

Adjunctive Therapy

The risk of recurrence after surgical pterygium removal has led to the addition of several physical or pharmacological therapies, the widest interest having been attracted in the recent years by mitomycin C. The effectiveness of any of these is balanced by the risk of complications. However, the limbal stem cell pathogenesis theory supports the use of cytotoxic therapies, because these would be able to eradicate the pterygium cells where surgery fails, as when they infiltrate normal-appearing tissue.

Radiation and Other Physical Therapies

Physical therapy is the oldest proposed adjunctive or even alternative method to treat pterygia, starting with cautery over 100 years ago.[44] The basic idea, common to cautery, β-radiation, and argon laser, is to inhibit new vessel formation. Angiogenesis undoubtedly plays a role in the scarring mechanism of recurrence. Nevertheless, the "collateral" damage to the altered epithelial cells could be the actual clue to their success.

According to the different series, β-radiation with strontium-90 reduces recurrences to an inter-

val between 1.7 and 13%,[45] or to about 1/3 to 1/4 of those occurring after surgery alone. However, the possible complications can be dreadful (scleral or corneal perforation, etc.) and may occur many years after treatment.

Interestingly, the use of an applicator of smaller size (3 by 8.5 mm) following the limbal curvature appears to reduce the risk of scleral necrosis.[46] This geometry actually favors the elimination of the limbal pterygium cells while minimizing the irradiation of the scleral bed.

Chemotherapy

The drugs most commonly used in conjunction with pterygium surgery are, of course, topical corticosteroids. In addition to anti-inflammatory effects, they may have direct antiangiogenic activity. The same property is sought with β-radiation and with thiotepa, the first antimitotic therapy used for this purpose.[4,31,47]

Although initially tried for pterygia in 1963,[48] mitomycin C only attained its current popularity after its success in glaucoma surgery. Mitomycin C is a more unspecific cytotoxic agent, with an activity spectrum beyond the proliferating vascular endothelial cell. This may explain its higher effectiveness in preventing recurrences compared to thiotepa. Nevertheless its primacy also relies in the simplicity of application, particularly with the single intraoperative dose[49] – a setting comparable to its success over 5-fluorouracil in filtering surgery.

Toxic complications inevitably accompany the use of potent drugs, and the literature of the recent years abounds in reports and controversies about the indications, dosages and complications of mitomycin C application in pterygium surgery.[33,50] The doses have been steadily reduced with no apparent loss of efficacy (mostly in the 5 to 8% recurrence rate) and an improvement in safety. However, corneoscleral meting has been reported even with a single intraoperative application at 0.02% for 3 minutes.[51] As is the case with β-radiation, the possibility of long-term complications calls for a careful approach and follow-up.

Current Approach

The usual clinical scenarios we encounter regarding pterygia fall into one of the following categories:

a Small and asymptomatic, or mildly symptomatic lesions, in a typically young and cosmetically concerned patient, or as an incidental finding in an older patient with other complaints.

b A symptomatic medium to large primary pterygium, causing recurrent irritative episodes, decreased vision, or an unbearable cosmetic blemish.

c A recurrent pterygium, causing increased disturbances and concern with successive surgical failures.

d A symptomatic or progressively growing limbal lesion, somewhat resembling a pterygium but lacking one or several of its defining features.

Adequate recognition of these situations, as well as an accurate diagnosis, excluding pseudopterygia, limbal tumors and other limbal diseases (especially in the "d" cases) are prerequisites for a successful management.

Small Primary Pterygia

In the first group (a), I usually try first preventive and medical measures, mostly based on nonpreserved artificial tears and blepharitis treatment when applicable. NSAI drops control most symptomatic episodes not responding to lubricants. Although steroids may have a faster and stronger effect, any lesion not responding to NSAI drops is probably becoming surgical. Vasoconstrictor drops will temporarily reduce redness and help the cosmetically concerned, but may lead to dependency and rebound effects.

In this type of case, if the patient demands surgery for cosmetic reasons or on the occasion of other (i.e., cataract) procedure, I use a *simple excision technique with primary closure*. These are small pterygia (even pingueculae) without risk factors for recurrence, so there is no need for grafts or adjunctive therapy. If the reason for surgery is recurrent irritation episodes not responding to medical treatment or a progressive growth of the lesion, these cases are reclassified into group (b).

My technique includes a head-first dissection with a Desmarres knife and pulling on the pterygium head with forceps. Once the head is detached from the cornea, the body is resected with Westcott scissors along horizontal or arcuate lines, slightly converging towards the inner canthus. There are usually no major attachments to the sclera and only some blunt dissection may be needed. Additional smaller cuts of 2-3 mm along the upper and lower limbus create "mini-flaps" for the conjunctival closure.

The corneal bed under the pterygium head is cleaned of scar tissue and regularized, also removing the surrounding epithelium for about 2 mm. The burr is seldom required in these cases. A coaxial bipolar diathermy probe with broad tip (eraser) is used to obtain a bloodless sclera without creating excessive burn. The eraser is also passed along the limbus, blanching not only the limbal arcades but also any remaining epithelium in the whole exposed sector, usually for about two clock hours. The conjunctiva is closed by direct apposition using one or two 8-0 vicryl sutures anchored to the sclera and leaving a bare zone of about 2 mm next to the limbus.

Medium to Large Primary Pterygia

Although medical therapy can be temporarily attempted, patients of group (b) usually require surgery. It is important to evaluate the risk factors for recurrence and to inform the patient accordingly, to insure his/her expectations will be realistic. Clinical risk factors for recurrence include: young age, present or past residence in low latitudes or desert climates, outdoor occupation, larger pterygium sizes, increased thickness or fleshiness,[4] and frequent recurrent inflammatory episodes.

In the absence of clear risk factors, my preferred surgical technique in these cases is *resection with conjunctival autograft*. I generally follow the technique of Kenyon et al.,[40] with few variations. When one or more risk factors are present, a sponge soaked in 0.02% mitomycin C is applied for 3 minutes on the scleral bed before placing the graft, followed by copious irrigation with saline.

The resection technique is similar to the one described in the previous section. Traction sutures may be necessary to mobilize adequately the globe. In case the scar tissue under the head is prominent, a diamond burr is used to regularize the corneal surface. The epithelium removal is extended to 3 mm around the bed and the limbus is erased for about a quadrant. The conjunctiva is obtained from the superior temporal quadrant of the same eye reaching the limbus, placed on the scleral bed maintaining the anatomic orientation but 1-mm posterior to the limbus, and fixated with 8-0 vicryl sutures. These will be removed one week later. Sliding the superior conjunctiva to about 1-2 mm from the limbus covers the donor site. In cases with particularly large pterygia or when the conjunctiva is not suitable due to previous surgery, scarring or other pathology, a mucous membrane graft form the lower lip is used as described below.

Recurrent and Multiple-Head Primary Pterygia

Recurrent pterygia, except in the case of very minor first recurrences, constitute generally a clear surgical indication. Primary cases with both nasal and temporal heads are considered in the same category. The preferred technique is in principle similar to the one used for a large single primary pterygium with risk factors: *resection, low-dose mitomycin C, and graft*. However, there may be multiple variations, and the operation must be planned carefully on an individualized basis.

The resection phase can be arduous, making it necessary to identify and protect the medial or other rectus muscles while the hypertrophic fibrovascular tissue and symblepharon are dissected. Although it is important to remove this excessive epibulbar or Tenon's tissue, care should be taken not to thin the sclera and to respect as much as possible of the superficial conjunctival layers not grossly involved. The excess scar under the pterygium head should be resected and burr polished, avoiding a deep keratectomy. It is not necessary to excise all opaque material but just to obtain a smooth surface, ideally at the original level of the corneal surface. It may be actually more important to remove, as in the above-described technique, a margin of corneal epithelium that may contain pterygium cells, even if normal-looking.

The nature of the graft required will vary according to the situation, as evaluated after the completion of the resection. If the total denuded scleral area is not greater than 12 by 12 mm, and the upper temporal conjunctiva appears normal, this can be used as the source for the graft. With any larger area, especially when the fornices have to be reconstructed, a buccal autograft is required. To obtain the mucous membrane, a clamp instrument is placed around the lower lip, stretching and everting it.

The mucosa is infiltrated with saline solution until the whole inner surface is smooth and taut. The Castroviejo electrokeratome with the 0.2-mm gauge plate is passed with a uniform movement. This allows the creation of a rectangular flap of about 15 by 40 mm.

The electrokeratome is removed and a metallic plate placed under the flap before the hinge is cut with scissors *(Figures 1-2 to 1-4)*. These grafts can be customized to fit one or multiple resection beds or to reconstruct the conjunctival fornices *(Figures 1-5 to 1-8)*.

In case there is significant thinning of the sclera and/or cornea, mitomycin C will not be used and a lamellar corneal or corneoscleral allograft is applied. We used to favor simple, circular lamellar corneal grafts either for the corneal alone *(Figures 1-9 to 1-12)* or covering both the corneal and scleral bed. More recently, corneoscleral allografts are preferred because of their limbus content.

CONCLUSION

The limbal stem cell theory of pterygium pathogenesis is changing the ways we understand and treat this puzzling pathology. The different mechanisms for primary and recurrent pterygia have to be taken into consideration. A primary pterygium is the result of altered limbal basal epithelial stem cells that become migratory (pterygium cells) and invade the cornea as an "advancing limbus", dragging a degenerated conjunctiva and further stimulating its hypertrophy and neovascularization by the release of cytokines such as TGF-β. It has to be understood that, contrary to other limbal disorders in which the limbal barrier is destroyed by the loss of the stem cells, allowing for the conjuntivalization of the cornea (as in alkali burns), here the altered stem cells are responsible for the invasion.

When this lesion is resected, recurrence may ensue either caused by: (a) remaining pterygium cells in the normal-appearing adjacent epithelium or the resection margins reinitiating the pathological process; (b) a hypertrophic scarring response of the remaining fibrovascular tissues or induced by the exposition of a large scleral bed; (c) unrecoverable loss of the limbal barrier leading to classical conjuntivalization of the cornea, or (d) a combination of these.

The goals of pterygium surgery must, therefore, include: (a) the eradication of all mutant pterygium cells; (b) the removal of all reactive fibrovascular tissue; (c) the restoration of a smooth surface, easy to re-epithelialize; and (d) the restoration of the normal limbal barrier.

While the first two require a meticulous resection (stressing the importance of the first goal over the second), the latter appear to be best served by the application of grafts. My experience with amniotic membrane is so far limited but promising, and I foresee a predominant role for it in the future.

The use of Mitomycin C or other adjunctive therapy may have a role in ensuring the eradication of pterygium cells and in suppressing the excessive scarring response if a safe and effective dosage is well established after a sufficient long term follow-up.

REFERENCES

1. Rosenthal JW. Chronology of pterygium therapy. *Am J Ophthalmol* 36:1601, 1953.

2. The American Heritage Dictionary of the English Language, Third Edition. Houghton Mifflin Company, 1992.

3. Youngson RM. Pterygium in Israel. *Am J Ophthalmol* 74:954, 1972.

4. Tan DTH, Chee S-P, Dear KBG, Lim ASM. Effect of pterygium morphology on pterygium recurrence in a controlled trial comparing conjunctival autografting with bare sclera excision. *Arch Ophthalmol* 115:1235, 1997.

5. Adamis AP, Starck T, Kenyon KR. The management of pterygium. *Ophthalmol Cin North Am* 3(4):611, 1990.

6. Oldenburg JB, Garbus J, McDonnell JM, McDonnell PJ. Conjunctival pterygia: mechanism of corneal topographic changes. *Cornea* 9:200, 1990.

7. Barraquer-Somers E, Chan CC, Green WE. Corneal epithelial iron deposition. *Ophthalmology* 90:729, 1983.

8. Ansari MW, Rahi AHS, Shukla BR. Pseudoelastic nature of pterygium. *Br J Ophthalmol* 54:473, 1970.

9. Austin P, Jakobiec FA, Iwamoto T. Elastodysplasia and elastodystrophy as the pathologic bases of ocular pterygia and pinguecula. *Ophthalmology* 90:96, 1983.

10. Kawano K, Uehara F, Ohba N. Lectin-cytochemical study on epithelial mucus glycoprotein of conjunctiva and pterygium. *Exp Eye Res* 47:43, 1888.

11. Cameron ME: Histology of pterygium: an electron microscopic study. *Br J Ophthalmol* 67:604, 1983.

12. Dushku N, Tyler N, Reid TW. Immunohistochemical evidence that pterygia arise from altered limbal epithelial basal stem cells. *Invest Ophthalmol Vis Sci* 34:1013, 1993.

13. Dushku N, Reid TW. Immunohistochemical evidence that human pterygia originate from an invasion of vimentin-expressing altered limbal epithelial basal cells. *Curr Eye Res* 13:473, 1994.

14. Dushku N, Reid TW. P53 expression in altered limbal basal cells of pingueculae, pterygia, and limbal tumors. *Curr Eye Res* 16:1179, 1997.

15. Talbot G. Pterygium. Trans Ohtalmol Soc NZ 2:42, 1948.

16. Cameron ME. Pterygium throughout the world. Springfield, IL, Charles C Thomas, 1965.

17. Goldberg L, David R. Pterygium and its relationship to the dry eye in the Bantu. *Br J Ophthalmol* 60:720, 1976.

18. McKenzie FD, Hirst LW, Battistutta D, Green A. Risk analysis in the development of pterygia. *Ophthalmology* 99:1056, 1992.

19. Threlfall TJ, English DR. Sun exposure and pterygium of the eye. A dose-response curve. *Am J Ophthalmol* 128:280, 1999.

20. Forsius H, Eriksson A. Pterygium and its relation to arcus senilis, pinguecula and other similar conditions. *Acta Ophthalmol* 40:402, 1962.

21. Hilgers JHC. Pterygium: Its incidence, heredity and etiology. *Am J Ophthalmol* 50:635, 1960.

22. Norn M, Franck C. Long-term changes in the outer part of the eye in welders. *Acta Ophthalmol* 69:382, 1991.

23. Scarpa A, cited by Poncet F. Du pterygion. *Arch Ophtalmol* (Paris) 1:21 1880-1881.

24. Detels R, Dhir SP: Pterygium. A geographical study. *Arch Ophthalmol* 78:485, 1967

25. Pinkerton OD, Hokama Y, Shigemura LA. Immunologic basis for the pathogenesis of pterygium. *Am J Ophthalmol* 98:225, 1984.

26. Barraquer JI. Etiología y etiopatogenia del pterigion y de las excavaciones en la córnea de Fuchs. *Arch Soc Am Oftal Optom* 5:45, 1964.

27. Miller D. Optical features of the ocular surface. Int Ophthalmol Clin 19(2):37-52, 1979.

28. Arenas E. Etiopatología de la pinguecula y el pterigio. *Pal Oftalmol Panam* 2(3):28-31, 1978.

29. Kwok LS, Coroneo MT. A model for pterygium formation. *Cornea* 13:219, 1994.

30. Levine AJ, Perry ME, Chang A, et al. The 1993 Walter Hubert lecture: The role of the p53 tumour-suppressor gene in tumorigenesis. *Br J Cancer* 69:409, 1994.

31. Dushku N, Hatcher SLS, Albert DM, Reid TW. p53 expression and relation to human papillomavirus infection in pingueculae, pterygia, and limbal tumors. *Arch Ophthalmol* 117:1593, 1999.

32. Jaros PA, DeLuise VP. Pingueculae and pterygia. *Surv Ophthalmol* 33:41, 1988.

33. Hoffman RS, Power WJ. Current options in pterygium management. *Int Ophthalmol Clin* 39(4):15-26, 1999.

34. Sugar HS. A surgical treatment for pterygium based on new concepts as to its nature. *Am J Ophthalmol* 32:912, 1949.

35. Krag S, Ehlers N. Excimer laser treatment of pterygium. *Acta Ophthalmol* 70:530, 1992.

36. Tseng SCG. Concept and application of limbal stem cells. Eye 3:141, 1989.

37. Tomas T. Sliding flap of conjunctival limbus to prevent recurrence of pterygium. *Refract Corneal Surg* 8:394, 1992.

38. Desmarres LA. Traité Théorique et Pratique des Maladies des Yeux, 2nd edition, vol 2, p 160. Paris, G Baillère, 1855.

39. Barraquer JI. Etiology, pathogenesis, and treatment of the pterygium. In: *Symposium on Medical and Surgical Diseases of the Cornea*, pp 167-178. Transactions of the New Orleans Academy of Ophthalmology. St Louis, CV Mosby, 1980.

40. Kenyon KR, Wagoner MD, Hettinger ME. Conjunctival autograft transplantation for advanced and recurrent pterygium. *Ophthalmology* 92: 1461, 1985.

41. Shimazaki J, Yang HY, Tsubota K. Limbal autograft transplantation for advanced and recurrent pterygia. *Ophthalmic Surg Lasers* 27:917, 1996.

42. Naumann GOH, Lang GK, Rummelt V, Wigand ME. Autologous nasal mucosa transplantation in severe bilateral conjunctival mucus deficiency syndrome. *Ophthalmology* 97:1011, 1990.

43. Kim JC, Tseng SCG. Transplantation of preserved human amniotic membrane for surface reconstruction in severely damaged rabbit corneas. Invest Ophthalmol Vis Sci 34(Suppl):1366, 1993.

44. Coe A. A new method of treating pterygium. *Ann Ophthalmol* 5:250, 1896.

45. Schultze J, Hinrichs M, Kimming B. Results of adjuvant radiation therapy after surgical excision of pterygium. *German J Ophthalmol* 5:207, 1996.

46. Levine DJ: Beta irradiation of pterygium. *Ophthalmology* 99:841, 1992.

47. Meacham R. Triethylene phosphoramide in the prevention of recurrent pterygium. *Am J Ophthalmol* 54:751, 1962.

48. Kunimoto N, Mori S. Studies on the pterygium. Part IV. A treatment of the pterygium by mitomycin C instillation. *Nippon Ganka Gakkai Zasshi* 67:601, 1963.

49. Frucht-Perry J, Islar M, Hemo I. Single dosage of mitomycin C for prevention of recurrent pterygium: preliminary report. *Cornea* 13:411, 1994.

50. Hardten DR, Samuelson TW. Ocular toxicity of Mitomycin-C. *Int Opthalmol Clin* 39(2):79, 1999.

51. Doughety PJ, Hardten DR, Lindstrom RL. Corneoscleral melt after pterygum surgery using a single intraoperative application of mitomycin-C. *Cornea* 15:537, 1996.

Ocular Surface Transplantation Techniques for Pterygium Surgery

Donald T.H. Tan, M.D.

Introduction

Cameron in 1972 stated that "Many surgeons consider the humble pterygium to be unworthy of their talents and sometimes for this reason, or under pressure of work, delegate the excision to junior staff, who in turn treat the condition in cavalier fashion, with, in some cases, poor results".[1] Unfortunately this is still true in many parts of the world today, and trivialisation of pterygium surgery, combined with inadequate surgical technique, are responsible for variable results and efficacy of excision procedures, leading to a general reluctance to perform surgery except in severe cases of central encroachment of the visual axis. Although in 1953 Rosenthal described a myriad of different surgical treatments for pterygium and reported that pterygia have been "incised, removed, split, transplanted, excised, cauterised, grafted, inverted, galvanised, heated, dissected, rotated, coagulated, repositioned and irradiated",[2] today pterygium surgery still varies from the simplest procedure of bare sclera excision, to complex and esoteric surgery such as lamellar keratoplasty and amniotic membrane transplantation. These procedures have a common goal, to both excise a pterygium and prevent its subse-

quent recurrence, and the fact that wide variations in techniques exist belies the unsatisfactory and inconsistent results often obtained. In addition, potentially blinding complications arising from adjunctive pterygium surgery are now well-recognised, and this has led to much discussion on the controversial issue of long term complications associated with such therapies.

Goal of Pterygium Surgery

Recurrence of pterygium regrowth onto the cornea after surgical excision is the single most common and frustrating cause of failure of pterygium surgery to both patient and surgeon, but recurrence rates reported in today's literature still vary widely from 2% to 89%.[3-5]

Focusing attention on the issue of postoperative pterygium recurrence has led to the development of new advances and techniques which are the focus of this chapter, which details advanced surgical techniques of ocular surface transplantation which provide important additions to the armamentarium of both the corneal surgeon and the comprehensive ophthalmologist.

OCULAR SURFACE TRANSPLANTATION SURGERY

In recent years, the concept of ocular surface disease (OSD) has arisen, in which disorders affecting the biological continuum of the ocular surface consisting of the corneal epithelium, conjunctiva tear film and eyelids, are grouped together as a distinct group of clinical entities. In the last decade, new surgical techniques of ocular surface transplantation have been described, and as pterygium is now recognised to represent a focal form of OSD arising from chronic environmental exposure of the ocular surface, new procedures for pterygium surgery are now available. With the advent of the modern conjunctival autograft transplant, a new standard for pterygium surgery in terms of both safety and efficacy has been attained, all other procedures today may benchmarked against this procedure. Conjunctival autografting has its disadvantages, however, as high recurrence rates occasionally reported may be related to the relative difficulty of this procedure, and to significant variance in technique which may influence graft success. A major problem with pterygium surgery has been its relative but almost universally low rate of financial remuneration, as compared to intraocular procedures such as cataract surgery, especially when one considers that a well-performed conjunctival autograft may take longer than phacoemulsification surgery. Combined with the fact that surgical skills of conjunctival surgery are significantly different from that of conventional intraocular surgery (and surgical training programs focus on the latter rather than the former), and that pterygium is a relatively uncommon condition in Western temperate climates, it is not surprising that there is a general deficiency in the development of essential surgical skills for good pterygium surgery.

OCULAR SURFACE TRANSPLANTATION PROCEDURES

The following ocular surface transplantion procedures are currently performed for pterygium surgery:

1. Conjunctival autograft transplantation
2. Conjunctival rotational autograft transplantation
3. Annular conjunctival autogaft transplantation
4. Limbal autograft transplantation
5. Amniotic membrane transplantation.

Along with the conjunctival autograft, newer modifications of the procedure have now been described, and these include the conjunctival rotational autograft and the annular conjunctival autograft. Recent identification of the corneal limbus as the source of limbal stem cells responsible for corneal epithelial cell maintenance has led to the development of limbal stem cell transplantation procedures such as limbal autograft transplantation and limbal allograft transplantation, and as focal limbal stem cell deficiency is a suggested aetiological hypothesis for a pterygium, limbal autografting has also been advocated.[6-8] Finally, transplantation of human amniotic membrane on the ocular surface as a basement membrane substrate to facilitate ocular surface healing and reepithelisation has been shown to reduce pterygium recurrence, and pterygium excision is now accepted as a major indication for amniotic membrane transplantation.

1. Conjunctival Autograft Transplantation

The use of a free conjunctival autograft to cover a bare sclera defect after pterygium excision was first described in 1931 by Gomez-Marquez, who utilised superior bulbar conjunctiva from the contralateral eye. Thoft is credited with the description of conjunctival transplantation as first form of ocular surface transplantation for unilateral ocular surface disease in 1977, but it was Kenyon, however, in 1985, who proposed the current conjunctival autograft transplantation technique for advanced and recurrent pterygium which is now considered to be the "gold standard" to which other procedures may be benchmarked.[9,10]

Conjunctival autograft transplantation is a form of ocular surface transplantation, whereby an autologous free conjunctival graft is obtained from the superior bulbar conjunctiva and sutured to the scleral bed after pterygium excision. The proce-

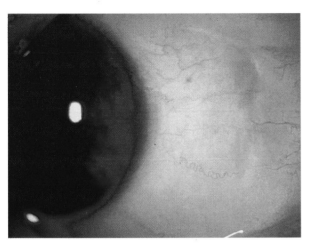

Figure 2-1. *Excellent cosmesis afforded by successful conjunctival autografting.*

	INDIVIDUAL SURGEONS' RECURRENCE RATE COMPARED TO PREVIOUS EXPERIENCE IN PERFORMING CONJUNCTIVAL AUTOGRAFTING	
Surgeon	No. of conjunctival autografts performed prior to study entry	Recurrence rate in study
A	10	5%
B	5	10%
C	4	14%
D	1	17%
E	1	30%
F-I	0	20-83%

dure has been shown to be safe, and effective, but is technically demanding. As a result, reported recurrence rates with conjunctival autografting vary considerably in the literature, from 2 to 35%.[3,5,10-12]

Conjunctival autografting was originally reserved for advanced or recurrent pterygium, but has now increasingly become accepted as the procedure of choice for a primary pterygium, due to the excellent cosmesis and low recurrence rate which can be achieved if correct surgical principles are maintained *(Figure 2-1)*. In 1994, we performed a randomised controlled trial in Singapore comparing conjunctival autografting with bare sclera excision

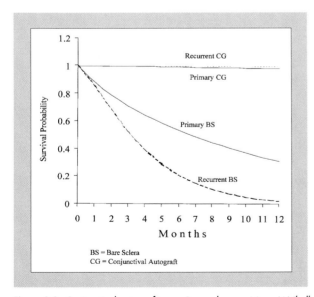

Figure 2-2. *Conjunctival autografting vs Bare sclera excision: Weibull survival curve analysis.*

for primary and recurrent pterygium. Results showed that conjunctival autografting could achieve a low recurrence rate (2%) in a tropical population in which the bare sclera recurrence rate was 61% for a primary pterygium, and 82% for a recurrent pterygium *(Figure 2-2)*.[3] However, this was a one surgeon efficacy trial, and analysis of conjunctival autografting among 23 surgeons in the same institution revealed a wide variation in recurrence rates ranging from 5% to 83%. In addition, there was a clear trend correlating prior surgical experience and study recurrence rate, with surgeons who had performed less autografts prior to study entry attaining higher recurrence rates. This suggests that conjunctival autografting is a relatively demanding procedure which has a significant learning curve, and may explain the range of recurrence rates reported in the literature.

Causes of Recurrence After Conjunctival Autografting

The morphological appearance of pterygium recurrence after conjunctival autografting suggests several factors, which may lead to graft failure. Recurrence of the pterygium may occur at the superior or inferior margins of the conjunctival graft, suggesting that either inadequate peripheral excision of pterygium tissue occurred, or insufficient graft size are contributing factors. A thick graft with inclusion of underlying Tenons tissue may lead to graft retraction and scalloping of the graft edge in the early postoperative period, causing exposure of bare sclera at the margins of the graft, which subsequently becomes the site of recurrence. Early breakage of sutures will also lead to localised graft retraction and localised recurrence at that site. However, it should be noted that in certain cases, a well-aligned and sutured, thin conjunctival graft may itself subsequently transform into a recurrent pterygium at the region of the limbus, suggesting that a corneal or limbal factor may be responsible for recurrence in this instance.

Essential Factors to Successful Conjunctival Autografting

Based on the mechanisms or recurrence associated with conjunctival autograft failure, important surgical principles may be inferred:

1. obtaining a large, generous graft (measuring 6 to 8 mm horizontally and vertically

2. adequate removal of all surrounding fibro-vascular tissue

3. obtaining a thin, Tenons-free graft (by superficial dissection techniques) to ensure minimal graft retraction

4. adequate stabilisation of graft with anchoring sutures at the limbus, superior and inferior edges of the graft.

Surgical Technique of Conjunctival Autografting

1. Pterygium Excision Technique

The aim is to ensure complete pterygium tissue removal without excessive tissue damage or scarring. Incomplete removal of remnant pterygium tissue may result in optical degradation of the precorneal tear film, while incomplete removal at the limbus and conjunctival aspects may increase the risk of pterygium recurrence. In addition, excessive tissue removal at the time or surgery may result in irregular astigmatism at the corneal aspect, and scleral thinning and dellen formation at the scleral bed. Excision of a recurrent pterygium is inherently more difficult as severe scarring obliterates tissue planes and there is therefore a higher

risk of extraocular muscle damage, and scleral or corneal tissue loss.

The principles of pterygium excision are:

1. complete removal of all pterygium tissue at Bowmans plane and the sclera

2. minimising scarring and astigmatism at the cornea

3. minimising scleral damage.

Anesthesia

Subconjunctival or regional anesthesia is sufficient in most instances. If additional surgery such as a conjunctival autograft is planned, retrobulbar or peribulbar anesthesia would be suitable options. General anesthesia may be indicated in exceptional cases of recurrent pterygium with marked muscle restriction and scarring.

Exposure/Stabilisation of the Globe

A corneal traction suture at the 12 o'clock limbus provides good traction to rotate the globe both horizontally during pterygium excision, and vertically during subsequent harvesting of a superior conjunctival autograft. A superior rectus bridle suture should be avoided in the latter instance as it may interfere with graft harvesting.

Excision of Pterygium Tissue

Pterygium fibers straddle across the cornea radially, and are most adherent at the limbus and at the pterygium head, but are minimally adherent to

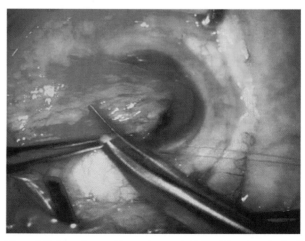

Figure 2-3. *Pterygium excision technique: initial incision site at body of pterygium.*

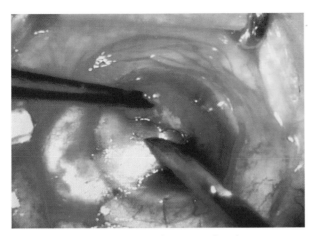

Figure 2-4. *Pterygium excision technique: Peeling / scraping pterygium tissue from Bowmans layer.*

the sclera, unless previous surgery has been performed. As such, a clean plane between pterygium tissue and underlying sclera is easily achieved if dissection is initiated at the scleral aspect, or body of the pterygium *(Figure 2-3)*. Care should be taken not to remove too much tissue, as horizontal tissue retraction occurs in all cases. Excision 3 to 4mm away from the limbus will result in an adequate bare sclera defect measuring 6 to 8 mm horizontally.

Reflection of the pterygium tissue towards the corneal aspect will expose limbal attachments, which may then be firmly detached using a #64 Beaver Microblade to scrape pterygium tissue from the sclera and limbus. It will now be possible to peel or scrape pterygium tissue off Bowmans layer

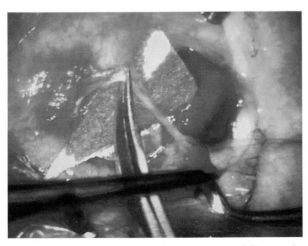

Figure 2-5. *Pterygium excision technique: removal of fibrovascular tissue by undermining of conjunctival edges.*

in a lamellar fashion *(Figure 2-4)*. Care should be taken to attempt to detach all pterygium tissue in one piece, which will reduce the risk of leaving remnant tissue tags on the cornea.

One should note that in some cases, a pterygium may be more deeply attached beyond Bowmans layer, and into the corneal stroma. Care should be taken to avoid deep dissection in these cases, which will result in excessive tissue loss.

All fibrovascular pterygium tissue should be removed at the scleral bed and limbus to reduce the risk of recurrence. A wide excision technique is therefore employed, necessitating removal of a thin strip of normal conjunctiva above and below the pterygium body.

Additional fibrovascular tissue may be removed at the conjunctival edges by exerting traction on subepithelial fibres and undermining the overlying conjunctival epithelium, but note that this will also result in further tissue retraction and a larger scleral bed defect *(Figure 2-5)*.

The role of the fibrovascular component of a pterygium in relation to surgical recurrence is demonstrated in the study by Tan and co-workers, in which recurrence after bare sclera excision was clearly found to be related to the degree of fibrovascular tissue in the pterygium.[3]

A clinical slit-lamp grading scale was developed, based on relative translucency of the body of the pterygium. Grade T1 (atrophic) denoted a pterygium in which episcleral vessels underlying the body of the pterygium were unobscured and clearly distinguished *(Figure 2-6a)*.

Grade T3 (fleshy) denoted a thick pterygium in which episcleral vessels underlying the body of the pterygium were totally obscured by fibrovascular tissue *(Figure 2-6c)*.

All other pterygia which did not fall into these 2 categories (i.e. episcleral vessel details were indistinctly seen or partially obscured) fell into Grade T2 (intermediate) *(Figure 2-6b)*. The study clearly showed that recurrence correlated well with translucency, with fleshy pterygium having the highest capacity for recurrence, while atrophic pterygium had the lowest.

The difference in recurrence rates were highly significant for both primary and recurrent pterygia *(Figures 2-7, 2-8)*.

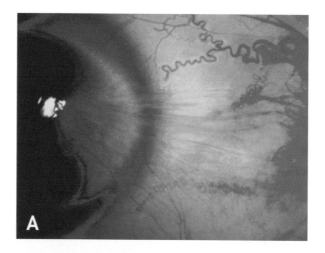

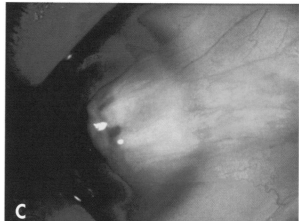

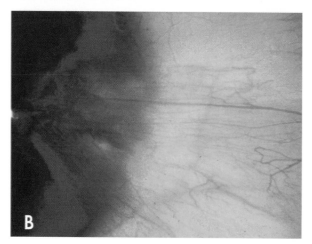

Figure 2-6. *Grading of Pterygium Morphology.*
A. *Grade T1: Atrophic Pterygium (episcleral vessels unobscured).*
B. *Grade T2: Intermediate Pterygium (episcleral vessels partially obscured).*
C. *Grade T3: Fleshy Pterygium (episcleral vessels totally obscured).*

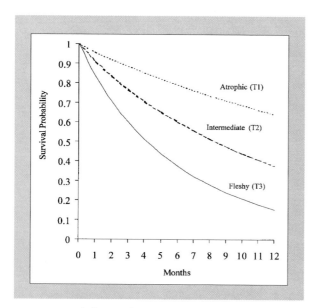

Figure 2-7. *Weibull Survival Curve Analysis - Primary Pterygia.*

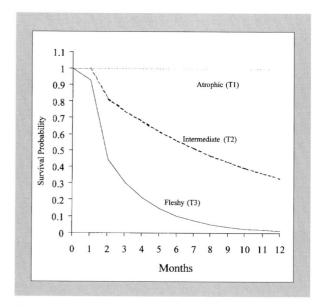

Figure 2-8. *Weibull Survival Curve Analysis - Recurrent Pterygia.*

Recurrent Pterygium Excision

Recurrent pterygium surgery should be performed by an experienced surgeon, as surgery is often difficult and hazardous. Previous surgery usually results in significant fibrous scarring and adherence to the underlying sclera throughout the body of the pterygium, with disortion of planes and landmarks. Adherence to corneal stroma will also be encountered if previous excision occurred deep to Bowmans layer. Loss of tissue planes make division of pterygium scar tissue from normal sclera and corneal stroma more difficult, and care should be taken to avoid an excessively deep dissection.

In many instances, the rectus muscle sheath may also be encased in the dense fibrous scar tissue. Occasionally, tractional forward migration of the insertion of the affected rectus muscle may occur, leading to the possibility of inadvertent damage or detachment of the muscle. Isolation of the involved rectus muscle posterior to the pterygium scar is therefore advised, prior to dissection of scar tissue, and all scar tissue around the muscle is required to prevent ocular motility restriction. Lid symblepharon, if present, should also be released, to allow the globe to fall back away from the eyelid.

2. Harvesting of the Conjunctival Autograft

An essential step to successful surgery is the careful harvesting of a thin, Tenon's free conjunctival autograft which is of adequate size. As it is this graft which is integral in the prevention of pterygium recurrence, a good surgical technique to harvest this autograft is needed to ensure a consistently low rate of recurrence when performing conjunctival autografting.

Harvesting Site

Upon completion of pterygium excision, the globe is rotated inferiorly to expose the superior bulbar conjunctiva which is the usual site for harvesting of the conjunctival graft (inferior bulbar conjunctiva may occasionally be utilised, but there may be inadequate tissue for a large graft, and inferior symblepharon with forniceal shortening may occur). A site far from the pterygium excision site is usually chosen, in order to leave a significant

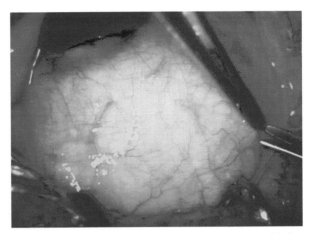

Figure 2-9. *Initial incision site for harvesting - superotemporal bulbar conjunctiva for a nasal pterygium.*

quadrant of untouched conjunctiva in the event of the need for future filtration surgery. For example, if a nasal pterygium is excised, the graft should be obtained from the superotemporal bulbar conjunctiva *(Figure 2-9)*.

Superficial Dissection Technique

An essential factor for success is to obtain a thin conjunctival graft. A natural tissue plane exists between Tenons layer and the episclera, and this is the usual deep plane for conjunctival dissection in filtration or strabismus surgery. However, no distinct tissue plane exists between Tenons layer and the conjunctival epithelium, and hence superficial dissection to separate these layers requires practice. A fine nick of the epithelial layer initially allows epithelium to be lifted up without inclusion of Tenons layer, and conjunctival scissors initiate the separation of the two layers. Careful lifting of the epithelium allows Tenons layer to be lifted and put on stretch, and Tenons fibers are cut close to the epithelium, allowing the subepithelial tissues to retract away *(Figures 2-10a, b)*. Blunt-tipped conjunctival forceps and scissors prevent inadvertent buttonholing of the graft, but a thinner graft may be obtained with fine-tipped scissors. Dissection is carried forward to the superior limbus.

This superficial dissection technique has the advantage of reducing conjunctival hemorrhage, and cautery is rarely needed. In addition, if Tenons layer is minimally disturbed, wound healing occurs

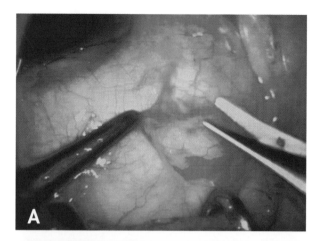

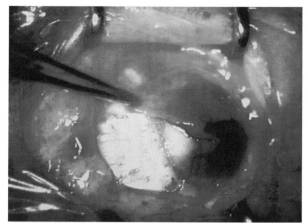

Figure 2-11. *Graft is carefully slid over from harvest site to recipient bed to maintain correct orientation.*

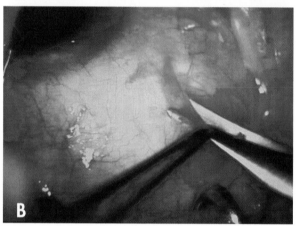

Figure 2-10. *Conjunctival autografting technique: graft harvesting technique.*
A. *Lifting of the epithelium allows Tenons layer to be stretched.*
B. *Tenons fibers are cut close to the epithelium, allowing the subepithelial tissues to retract away.*

without significant conjunctival scarring, and it is possible to reharvest conjunctiva from the same site.

Size of Conjunctival Autograft

Despite superficial dissection, some graft retraction will still occur as it is not possible to exclude subepithelial fibrous tissue completely. One should therefore aim to oversize the graft in relation to the donor site by at least 1 mm in each diameter. Initially, careful measurement and marking of recipient bed and donor is useful to assist in accurate graft and scleral bed proportions.

Orientation of Conjunctival Autograft

Although the theory of transplanting limbal stem cells by maximising inclusion of limbal epi-

thelium is attractive, no evidence exists that superficial conjunctival dissection is capable of including deep-lying limbal stem cells within the graft, and clinically, anatomical limbus-to-limbus orientation of the graft does not appear to be essential for graft success. However, it is essential that the conjunctival graft is correctly positioned with the epithelium uppermost, and it is recommended that upon completion of the harvesting, the graft is carefully slid into place from the superior harvest site to the bare sclera bed *(Figure 2-11)*. Inadvertent inversion of the graft will result in rapid desloughing in the early postoperative period.

Securing the Conjunctival Autograft

The conjunctival autograft is secured in place with interrupted sutures. 10-0 Vicryl or 8-0 virgin silk sutures are preferred. Initial suture placement should involve the limbal limits of the graft, followed by the superior and inferior edges of the graft *(Figures 2-12a-c)*. It is important that the graft is sutured to underlying episclera over these sites, to prevent graft displacement during ocular movements. Suturing of the graft overlying the rectus muscle should not include underlying muscle tissue. Finally, a central limbal suture is also necessary to prevent forward migration, or bowstringing, of the graft onto the cornea *(Figure 2-12d)*. A subconjunctival antibiotic/steroid injection completes the procedure. A final check should be made to ensure that the graft remains well se-

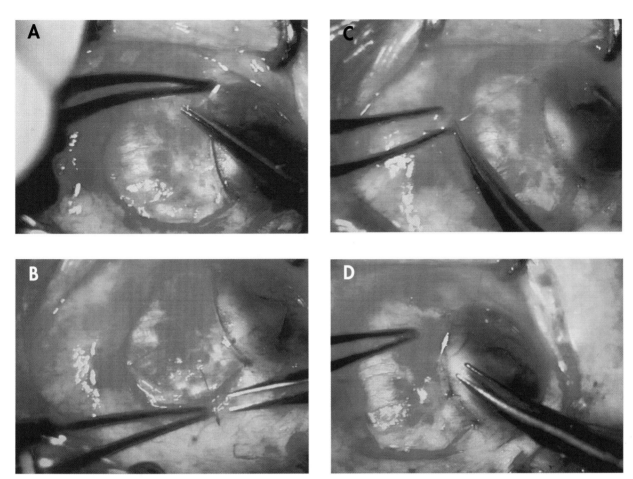

Figure 2-12. *Conjunctival autografting technique: suturing technique.*
A. *Initial suture placement should involve the limbal limits of the graft.*
B. *Upper and lower limits of graft should be sutured to episclera.*
C. *Suturing of canthal limit of graft should be limited to superficial conjunctiva, to avoid rectus muscle involvement.*
D. *Final central limbal sutures should be placed to prevent bowstringing of the graft across the limbus.*

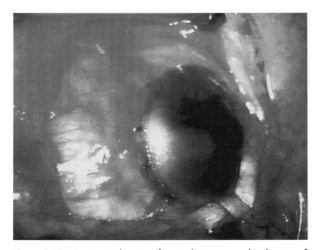

Figure 2-13. *Conjunctival autografting technique: completed autograft firmly secured in place on the globe.*

cured to the globe despite rotation of the eye *(Figure 2-13)*.

Additional techniques

Subconjunctival injection of anesthetic over the harvest site may assist in dissection as the conjunctival epithelium is theoretically ballooned away from subepithelial tissue. However, injection fluid follows the path of least resistance, and often fluid migrates inferiorly, ballooning Tenons layer as well, making superficial dissection more difficult.

Deliberate cuts within the graft at the end of the procedure are aimed at reduction of postoperative graft oedema by providing drainage sites for oedema fluid to escape. However, these cuts rapidly re-epithelise within days of surgery, and oedema re-accumulates.

Postoperative Regime

Topical steroid/antibiotic eyedrops are usually required for a month after surgery, as significant ocular surface inflammation occurs with conjunctival autografting. Care should be taken to identify steroid responders during this period. Graft oedema occurs to some degree in all cases, and should only be a cause of concern if severe enough to cause adjacent corneal dellen formation. Graft hemorrhage may also occur, and drainage or clot removal may be indicated in rare instances of severe hemorrhage. Premature suture breakage with localised graft retraction requires resuturing, as localise pterygium recurrence will occur.

Variants of Conjunctival Autografting

Certain situations may not permit conventional conjunctival autografting to be performed. As an integral part of the procedure is to obtain healthy tissue from the superior bulbar conjunctiva, eyes with prior damage or scarring in that area may make harvesting of tissue impossible. In addition, in cases in which several quadrants of limbus are involved, for example, broad pterygia, or combined medial and temporal pterygia, conventional autografting may not be feasible. In these situations the modified techniques of conjunctival rotational autografting and annular conjunctival autografting are required. Note these procedures are more advanced forms of conjunctival autografting, only to be attempted after mastering conventional conjunctival autografting.

2. Conjunctival Rotational Autografting

The major disadvantage of conjunctival autografting lies in the fact that harvesting a graft from the superior bulbar conjunctiva inevitably results in further ocular surface surgery in an eye with an already existing focal ocular surface disorder. In certain situations, surgery involving superior bulbar conjunctiva is contraindicated, or not possible. These situations include glaucoma patients with pre-existing drainage surgery blebs or seton surgery, glaucoma patients in which glaucoma surgery may possibly be indicated in future, or pre-existing scarring in which harvesting a thin conjunctival graft would be very difficult. Alternatively, in cases in which excessively large or several grafts are required, for example in combined nasal and temporal ptergium surgery, or in combined cataract and pterygium surgery, it may be undesirable to have a large conjunctival defect adjacent to a limbal cataract incision, conventional autografting may not be ideal.

We have described a modified procedure of conventional autografting, in which superior bulbar conjunctiva need not be utilised, which is termed conjunctival rotational autografting.[13] In this technique, conjunctival epithelium overlying the pterygium itself is carefully dissected, and laid aside. After removal of the underlying fibrovascular pterygium tissue, this epithelium is relaid over the bare sclera after a 180 degree rotation so that nasal canthal epithelium is now applied to the limbal area *(Figures 2-14a-d)*.

A "rotated island graft" was first described by Spaeth in the 1920s.[14] Blatt in 1931 suggested that a 180 degree rotation of the graft displaces abnormal epithelium at the head of the pterygium away from the limbus, which in turn receives relatively normal epithelium from the nasal canthus.[15]

Our prospective single surgeon case series of 51 consecutive rotational autografts for 46 primary and 5 recurrent pterygia revealed a recurrence rate of 4% at a mean follow-up period of 12 months (range 2-22 months), suggesting that the efficacy of this procedure in reducing recurrence may be similar to that of conventional conjunctival autografting.[13] Indications for rotational autografting in this series included glaucoma patients, superior conjunctival scarring, simultaneous nasal and temporal pterygium surgery, and combined cataract and pterygium surgery.

It should be noted, however, that rotational autografting is significantly more difficult to perform, as thin dissection of pterygium epithelium, with separation of underlying pterygium fibrovascular tissue, is difficult. In addition, oversizing of the graft is not possible. As such conjunctival rotational autografting should only be attempted by surgeons who are already skilled in conventional

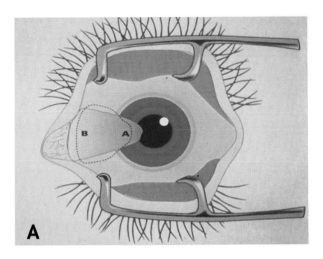
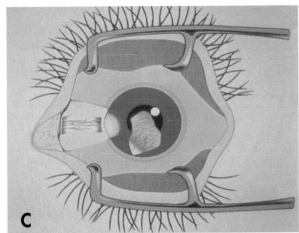
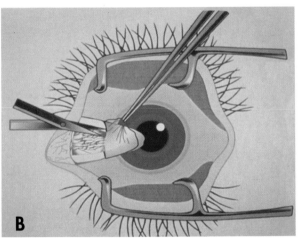
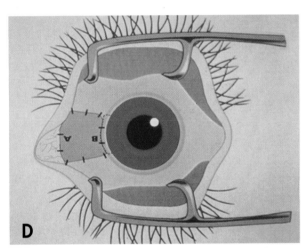

Figure 2-14. *Conjunctival rotational autograft.*
A. *The area of conjunctival epithelium to be harvested is outlined by the black dotted line. "A" represents the edge of the graft nearest the pterygium head, and "B" the edge nearest the canthus.*
B. *The epithelial layer (with minimal subepithelial tissue) is dissected free taking care not to include the underlying fibrovascular pterygium tissue.*
C. *The epithelial layer is laid aside, while underlying fibrovascular pterygium tissue is excised.*
D. *The epithelial layer is replaced with a 180 degree reorientation onto the bared scleral bed (epithelial surface up).*

conjunctival autografting. Other disadvantages of this procedure are prolonged graft hyperemia in some cases, and increased epithelial pigmentation in highly pigmented conjunctiva. However, in the majority of cases, rotational autografting may achieve excellent cosmesis, if properly performed *(Figures 2-15a-c).*

3. Annular Conjunctival Autografting

In extreme cases of severe pterygium encroachment of the cornea, two or more quadrants of limbus may be destroyed by fibrovascular pterygium invasion. In cases of severe combined nasal and temporal pterygium, close proximity of lesions either superiorly or inferiorly result in virtual merging of pterygia which again involves a large area of limbus. In these instances, the conventional technique of graft harvesting in conjunctival autografting will be inadequate to cover the subtotal limbal defect.

We have therefore described a modification of conjunctival autografting, whereby an elongated segment of conjunctiva is applied to the limbus to ensure full coverage of the annular limbal defect.[16] To obtain an elongated strip of conjunctiva, a large conventionally-shaped rectangular graft is first harvested from the superior bulbar conjunctiva.

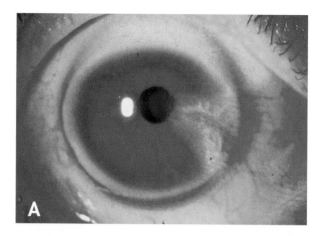

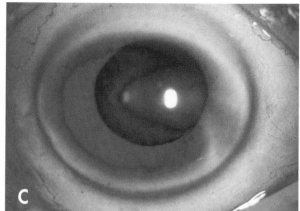

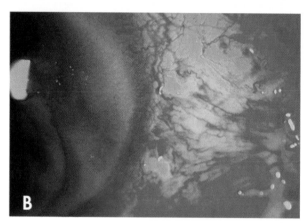

Figure 2-15. Conjunctival rotational autograft in a patient with pterygium and pre-existing glaucoma.
A. Preoperative state.
B. Nine days after pterygium excision with rotational autografting.
C. Seventeen months after surgery.

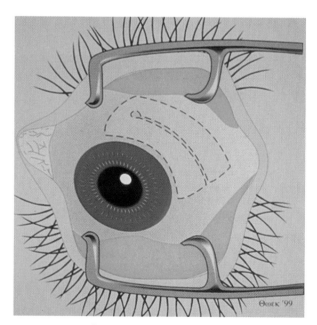

Figure 2-16. Annular conjunctival autografting: a larger graft from the superior bulbar conjunctiva is partially divided lengthwise to obtain an elongated strip of conjunctiva.

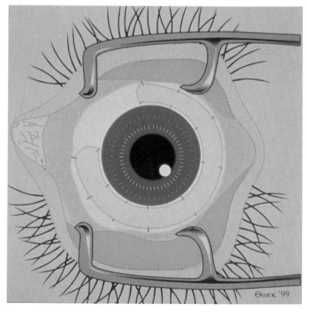

Figure 2-17. Annular conjunctival autografting: the elongated strip of conjunctiva is wrapped around the limbal defect.

136

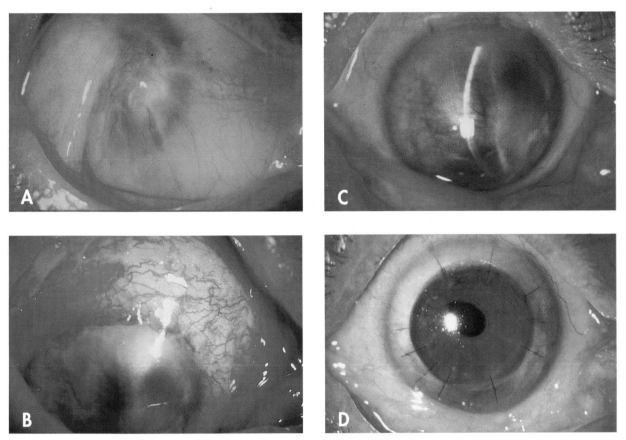

Figure 2-18. *Annular conjunctival graft in a patient with advanced subtotal pterygium.*
A. *Pre-operative state.*
B. *Seven days after surgery B the elongated strip is in place around the limbus.*
C. *Successful annular conjunctival autografting 6 months after surgery - no recurrence noted.*
D. *Two years after penetrating keratoplasty: no pterygium recurrence is noted.*

This graft is then partially divided in its long axis to form a enlongated strip *(Figure 2-16)*. This may now be carefully wrapped around the limbus to cover the scleral defect and sutured in place *(Figure 2-17)*.

Figures 2-18a-c illustrate the successful implementation of annular conjunctival autografting in an advanced pterygium involving most of the cornea and limbus *(Figure 2-18a)*.

The elongated strip of conjunctiva is clearly seen 1 week after surgery *(Figure 2-18b)*. Six months after pterygium surgery, no recurrence was noted, and the patient subsequently underwent successful penetrating keratoplasty *(Figures 2-18c, 2-18d)*.

4. Limbal Autograft Transplantation

Focal or partial limbal deficiency is a recent theory of pterygium aetiology in which excessive chronic sunlight or ultraviolet light exposure is hypothesized to damage limbal stem cells in the interpalpebral limbus, leading to conjunctiva-lisation of the nasal or temporal conjunctiva.

The finding of abnormal accumulation or over-expression of the tumour suppressor gene p53 supports this theory, in that UV irradiation is known to induce p53 mutations, and chronic UV exposure is a known epidemiological risk factor, and a pterygium is now considered by many to be a disorder of abnormal growth, as opposed to a simple degenerative process. If UV-induced limbal stem cell deficiency is responsible, then focal replacement of limbus is a reasonable, and limbal autograft transplantation for pterygium has been advocated by Shimazaki.[17] In fact, some argue that conjunctival autografting inadvertently transplants limbal stem cells from the superior limbus, accounting for the success of the procedure, and advocate correct anatomical apposition of limbal conjunctiva to the host limbus when performing a conjunctival autograft. In our experience, however, rotation of the autograft to fit the bare sclera defect (such that the conjunctival limbal area is no longer opposed to the host limbal bed) does not appear to increase recurrence rates, and as limbal stem cells are deeply situated in the limbus, it is not known if any limbal stem cells are transplanted at all when conventional conjunctival harvesting is performed. No appropriate randomised controlled trials have been performed to compare the relative efficacy of conjunctival autografting and limbal autografting and as very low rates of recurrence occur can be achieved with conventional autografting, it is unlikely that such a trial, if performed, will yield significant differences between the two procedures. Limbal autografting, while able to achieve low recurrence rates, should perhaps be reserved for cases of limbal stem cell failure from multiple previous ptergyium procedures, and/or the use of adjunctive therapy such as Mitomycin C ar beta-irradiation.

5. Amniotic Membrane Transplantation

Human amniotic membrane has been utilised in surgery since the 1940s, and its basement membrane properties have been shown to facilitate epithelialization and reduce scarring. In 1995, Kim and Tseng first reported on the ophthalmic use of amniotic membrane transplantation (AMT) to reconstruct the ocular surface in a rabbit chemical burn model, and since then, several reports have been published on the successful use of AMT for ocular surface reconstruction.[18] Tsubota et al combined AMT with limbal allograft transplantation to reconstruct the surface in patients with ocular cicatricial pemphigoid and Stevens Johnson syndrome, while AMT has also been utilised to treat chemical and thermal burns in combination with limbal transplantation.[19,20]

Cryopreserved human amniotic membrane for ocular surface transplantation is now available from a handful of eye or tissue banks.

Tseng has advocated that the ability of human amniotic membrane to facilitate re-epithelisation, reduce inflammation, scarring and vascularisation lends itself to pterygium surgery, as the phenomenon of pterygium recurrence itself probably involves recurrence of inflammatory processes, scarring and fibrosis and revascularisation of the conjunctiva, limbus and cornea. Tseng and co-workers performed amniotic membrane transplantation for pterygium surgery, and published a randomised controlled trial comparing excision with simple primary closure, conjunctival autografting and amniotic membrane transplantation.[12] Study results revealed recurrence rates of 45%, 4.9% and 14.8% for these respective procedures, establishing that although AMT was not able to match the success of conjunctival autografting, AMT indeed significantly reduces pterygium recurrence, as compared to simple excision procedures. Clinical results of AMT are also now supported by laboratory studies on the properties of AMT. Fukuda and co-workers evaluated the distribution of subchains of type IV collagen and laminin in amniotic membrane and compared this with corneal and conjunctival tissues.[21] Results showed that the distribution of subchains of type IV collagen in amniotic membrane were identical to that in the conjunctiva, but different from that in the cornea, suggesting that amniotic membrane is a useful replacement for conjunctiva, based on their shared basement membrane properties.

A major advantage of amniotic membrane transplantation over conventional autografting is that it is unnecessary to harvest a free conjunctival graft from superior conjunctiva, and hence, may be reserved for cases for which conventional autografting is contraindicated or difficult. As such, the indications for AMT are similar to that of conjunctival rotational autografting - AMT is simpler to perform, but is limited by the availability of amniotic membrane from a tissue bank. Figures 2-19a-e show an example of successful AMT surgery for pterygium - note the excellent cosmetic appearance which may be achieved by the amniotic membrane, presumably a result of its anti-inflammatory and anti-fibrotic qualities.

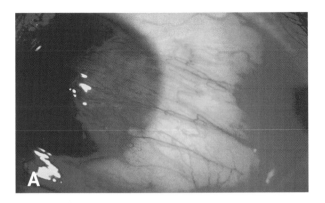

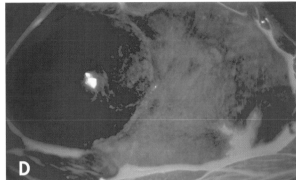

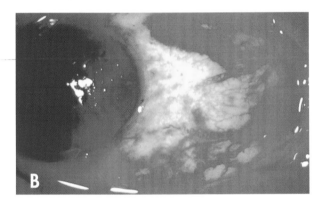

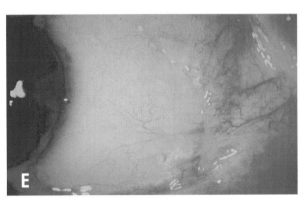

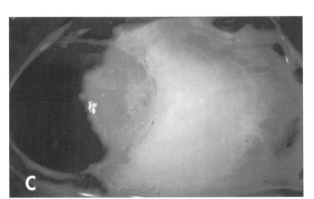

Figure 2-19. *Amniotic Membrane Transplantation for primary pterygium.*

A. *Preoperative state.*

B. *1ˢᵗ postoperative day - Amniotic membrane firmly in place over bare scleral bed.*

C. *1ˢᵗ postoperative day - Fluorescein stains both the corneal epithelial defect and the amniotic membrane which has yet to undergo epithelisation.*

D. *7ᵗʰ postoperative day - Minimal fluorescein staining of the amniotic membrane reveals that the surface is almost fully epithelised.*

E. *6 months after surgery reveals an excellent cosmetic result, no recurrence or residual ocular surface inflammation at the site of amniotic membrane placement.*

Surgical Technique of Amniotic Membrane Transplantation

Amniotic membrane transplantation is a relatively simpler procedure than conjunctival autografting, as harvesting a free conjunctival graft is unnecessary. However, there are some essential points to note when performing AMT surgery:

Size of Amniotic Membrane Graft

As amniotic membranes supplied by eye or tissue banks are often large in size, it is possible to remove significantly greater amounts of pterygium epithelial and fibrovascular tissue as compared to conventional conjunctival autografting. In addition, as some degree of re-encroachment of pterygium fibrovascular tissue usually occurs at the edges of the amniotic graft, it is usually advisable to place amniotic membrane tissue up to the canthal area. In general the size of an amniotic membrane graft is 50% to 100% larger than a conjunctival autograft which is limited by the size of the graft obtained from the superior conjunctiva.

Scleral bed preparation

As with conjunctival autografting, it is essential to remove as much fibrovascular pterygium tissue from the scleral bed as possible before applying the membrane. Careful haemostasis of the scleral bed is also essential, as postoperative haemorrhage beneath an amniotic membrane graft can persist for several weeks, and we have noted that focal recurrence of pterygium tissue may occur at the site of haemorrhage.

Amniotic membrane application

Amniotic membrane should be laid down with its smooth, non-sticky surface (epithelial side up) facing up, to enable rapid epithelisation of the membrane surface by conjunctival epithelium. The graft should be sutured in place under gentle traction with interrupted 10/0 monofilament Vicryl sutures, which should approximate membrane to peripheral conjunctiva. Inadequate tension will result in a "baggy", sagging graft which will impede re-epithelisation, while excessive graft tension will result in inward scalloping of the graft edges in-between sutures, leading to a smaller graft area.

Postoperative Management

As with conjunctival autografting, postoperative steroid and antibiotic eyedrops will be required for the first few weeks after surgery. The graft should be examined weekly to monitor the progress of graft epithelisation, which is usually complete by 2 weeks. It should be noted that, similar to conjunctival autografting, pterygium recurrence may still occur several months later and patients should either be followed up for at least 6 months after surgery, or return upon early signs of pterygium recurrence.

Summary

The acquisition of surgical skills and principles of fine conjunctival surgery are essential prerequisites for successful pterygium surgery with a low recurrence rate and good cosmesis. A variety of new conjunctival transplantation techniques are now available to achieve this, and these include conjunctival autograft transplantation, rotational conjunctival autografting, annular conjunctival autografting and amniotic membrane transplantation. Utilisation of these techniques provide a satisfactory alternative to antimitotic adjunctive therapies, with their attendant longterm risks and complications.

References

1. Cameron ME. Preventable complications of pterygium excision with beta-irradiation. *British Journal of Ophthalmology* 1972; 56: 52-56.

2. Rosenthal JW. Chronology of pterygium therapy. *American Journal of Ophthalmology* 1953; 36: 1601-1616.

3. Tan DTH, Chee SP, Dear KBG, Lim ASM. Effect of pterygium morphology on pterygium recurrence in a controlled trial comparing conjunctival autografting with bare sclera excision. *Archives of Ophthalmology* 1997; 115: 1235-1240.

4. Singh G, Wilson MR, Foster CS. Mitomycin eye drops as treatment for pterygium. *Ophthalmology* 1988; 95: 813-821.

5. Chen PP, Ariyasu RG, Kaza V, LaBree LD, McDonnell PJ. A randomized trial comparing mitomycin C and conjunctival autograft after excision of primary pterygium. *American Journal of Ophthalmology* 1995; 120.2: 151-160.

6. Tseng SCG, Tsai RJ-F. Limbal transplantation for ocular surface reconstruction - a review. *Fortschr Ophthalmol* 1991; 88: 236-242.

7. Tan DTH, Ficker LA, Buckley RJ. Limbal transplantation. *Ophthalmology* 1996; 103.1: 29-36.

8. Tan DTH, Lim ASM, Goh HS, Smith DR. Abnormal expression of the p53 tumor suppressor gene in the conjunctiva of patients with pterygium. *American Journal of Ophthalmology* 1997; 123.3: 404-405.

9. Thoft RA. Conjunctival transplantation. *Archives of Ophthalmology* 1977; 95: 1425-1427.

10. Kenyon KR, Wagoner MD, Hettinger ME. Conjunctival autograft transplantation for advanced and recurrent pterygium. *Ophthalmology* 1985; 92.11: 1461-1470.

11. Lewallen S. A randomized trial of conjunctival autografting for pterygium in the topics. *Ophthalmology* 1989; 96.11: 1612-1614.

12. Prabhasawat P, Barton K, Burkett G, Tseng SCG. Comparison of conjunctival autografts, amniotic membrane grafts, and primary closure for pterygium excision. *Ophthalmology* 1997; 104.6: 974-985.

13. Jap A, Chan C, Lim L, Tan DTH. Conjunctival rotation

autograft for pterygium. *Ophthalmology* 1999; 106.1: 67-71.

14. Spaeth ED. Rotated island graft operation for pterygium. *American Journal of Ophthalmology* 1926; 9: 649-655.

15. Blatt N. Replantation of pterygium as a method of operation for pterygium. Ztschr.f.Augenh. 1932; 76: 161

16. Yip CC, Lim L, Tan DTH. The surgical management of an advanced pterygium involving the entire cornea. *Cornea* 1997; 16.3: 365-368.

17. Shimazaki J, Yang H-Y, Tsubota K. Limbal autograft transplantation for recurrent and advanced pterygia. *Ophthalmic Surgery and Lasers* 1996; 27.11: 917-923.

18. Kim JC, Tseng SCG. Transplantation of preserved human amniotic membrane for surface reconstruction in severely damaged rabbit corneas. *Cornea* 1995; 14.5: 473-484.

19. Tsubota K, Satake Y, Ohyama M. Surgical reconstruction of the ocular surface in advanced ocular cicatricial pemphigoid and Stevens-Johnson syndrome. *American Journal of Ophthalmology* 1996; 122: 38-52.

20. Shimazaki J, Yang H-Y, Tsubota K. Amniotic membrane transplantation for ocular surface reconstruction in patients with chemical and thermal burns. *Ophthalmology* 1997; 104.12: 2068-2076.

21. Fukuda.Ken, Chikama T, Nakamura M, Nishida T. Differential distribution of subchains of the basement membrane components Type IV collagen and laminin among the amniotic membrane, cornea, and conjunctiva. *Cornea* 1999; 18.1: 73-79.

3

AMNIOTIC MEMBRANE TRANSPLANTATION IN PTERYGIUM SURGERY

Abraham Solomon, M.D. — Scheffer C.G. Tseng, M.D., Ph.D.

BACKGROUND

Introduction

The three main goals of pterygium surgery are to prevent recurrence, to achieve an acceptable cosmetic result, and to avoid complications. Although many surgical methods were developed to excise the lesion, to cover the defect, and to prevent recurrence with adjunctive treatments, none has offered recurrence-free results. The various adjunctive treatments, such as beta irradiation, thio-thepa, and mitomycin C are associated with numerous side effects. Conjunctival autograft to cover the defect is currently the method associated with the least recurrence rate. However it is difficult to cover large areas in cases of a double-head pterygium or an advanced pterygium with a wide conjunctival involvement. Furthermore, removal of a free conjunctival graft may not be possible in a previously operated eye with scarring, and may present a problem for glaucoma-filtering surgery in the future. These considerations have led to the inclusion of amniotic membrane transplantation as a method of covering the defect following the removal of pterygium.

The Amniotic Membrane in Ocular Surface Surgery

Amniotic membrane, or amnion, is the innermost layer of the placenta. It consists of a thick basement membrane and an avascular stromal matrix *(Figure 3-1, right)*. Amniotic membrane transplantation has been described for reconstruction in different medical subspecialties in the early literature (for review see [1]).

In the English literature, a live fetal membrane including both amnion and chorion was first used with a limited success by De Rotth[2] in 1940 as a graft for symblepharon lysis. Sorsby et al[3,4] in 1946 and 1947 reported the use of chemically-processed dry amniotic membrane as a patch for treating acute ocular burns.

For reasons still not clear, the use of the amniotic membrane disappeared from the literature until 1995 when Kim and Tseng[5] reintroduced it for treating corneal surfaces with limbal stem cell deficiency. Since then this procedures have been reported for various ophthalmic uses. When appropriately processed and preserved, the amniotic membrane can be used in a number of indications, whether as a graft to replace the damaged ocular

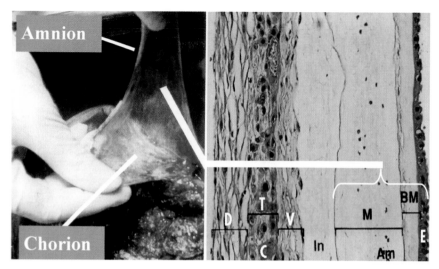

Figure 3-1

Right: *Histologic section of a human placenta, showing its different layers.*
C = *chorion*
Am = *amniotic membrane*
M = *amniotic stromal matrix*
BM = *basement membrane*
E = *epithelium*
D = *decidua*
T = *trophoblast*
V = *villus*
In = *the space potentially present between the amnion and the chorion. Note the thick avascular matrix of the amniotic membrane.*

Left: *Manual dissection of the amniotic membrane from the human placenta from the space (In). The amniotic membrane can easily be separated from the chorion.*

surface stromal matrix, or as a patch to prevent unwanted inflammatory insults from gaining access to the damaged ocular surface.

Amniotic membrane transplantation has been used for the past several years for conjunctival surface reconstruction in order to restore a normal stroma and to provide a healthy basement membrane for renewed epithelial proliferation and differentiation. Specifically, it has been used to reconstruct the conjunctival surface as an alternative to conjunctival graft following removal of large conjunctival lesions such as a pterygium,[6,7] conjunctival intraepithelial neoplasia and tumors,[8] scars and symblepharon,[8,9] and conjunctivochalasis.[8] These reports indicate that the reconstructed area can be very large so long as the underlying bed is not ischemic and the bordered conjunctiva has a normal epithelium and subconjunctival stroma.

Action Mechanisms of the Amniotic Membrane

Following the removal of a pterygium, the remaining bare sclera is denuded of a basement membrane. If healing is allowed to take place on a large defect, scar tissue or granuloma may develop. Scarring can result in annoying redness, irritation, symblepharon formation, and motility restriction. Therefore, there is a need to facilitate rapid epithelialization so that tear-derived inflammation can be

impeded. The basement membrane is known to facilitate migration,[10] reinforce adhesion,[11,12] promote differentiation,[13-16] and prevent apoptosis[17,18] of epithelial cells. Therefore one action mechanism of the amniotic membrane is to promote the healing of epithelial cells, an action consistent with the report that amniotic membrane can promote epithelialization for persistent corneal epithelial defects with stromal ulceration.[19-21]

The amniotic membrane can also promote nongoblet cell differentiation of the conjunctival epithelium.[22]

Conjunctival goblet cell differentiation is further promoted by coculturing with conjunctival fibroblasts on the same side of the basement membrane.[23] This data supports the fact that conjunctival goblet cell density is promoted following amniotic membrane transplantation in vivo.[24]

In addition to these effects, which are associated with the basement membrane side, the stromal side of the membrane has other attributes. The stromal side of the membrane contains a unique matrix component that suppresses TGF-b signaling, proliferation and myofibroblast differentiation of normal human corneal and limbal fibroblasts.[25] This action explains why amniotic membrane transplantation helps in reducing scars during conjunctival surface reconstruction,[8] preventing recurrent scarring after pterygium removal,[6] and reducing corneal haze following PTK and PRK.[26,27] Although such an action is more potent when fibroblasts are in contact with the stromal matrix, a lesser effect is also noted when fibroblasts are separated from the membrane by a distance, suggesting that some diffusible factors might also be involved besides the insoluble matrix components in the membrane. In line with this thinking, several growth factors have been identified in the amniotic membrane.[28] The stromal matrix of the membrane can also exclude inflammatory cells by rendering them into rapid apoptosis,[26,29] and contains various forms of protease inhibitors.[30] This action explains why stromal inflammation is reduced after amniotic membrane transplantation[8,19] and corneal neovascularization is mitigated,[31] actions important for preparing the stroma for supporting limbal stem cells to be transplanted either at the same time or later.[7,32-34] This action also explains why keratocyte apoptosis can be reduced and hence the stromal haze is prevented in PRK or PTK by amniotic membrane. [26,29,35]

The anti-inflammatory property of the amniotic membrane is of special importance in dealing with pterygium fibroblasts. These fibroblasts have a transformed phenotype and thus may overexpress certain matrix-degrading enzymes in response to pro-inflammatory cytokines that are derived from the ocular surface. Specifically, we had demonstrated an increased expression of MMP-1 and-3 by pterygium body fibroblasts in response to their stimulation with interleukin-1β or tumor necrosis factor α[36]. Therefore, the presence of the amniotic membrane in the vicinity of activated pterygium fibroblasts that remain as a result of incomplete tissue removal may have an added beneficial effect. By decreasing inflammatory stimuli, further activation of residual pterygium fibroblasts is prevented, thus reducing the risk of fibrovascular proliferation and subsequent recurrence.

SURGICAL TECHNIQUE

Preparation of the Amniotic Membrane

Careful preparation and preservation of the amniotic membrane are important to assure successful results.[8,19,34] Human placenta is obtained from an elective cesarean section, from seronegative donors for human immundeficiency virus (HIV), hepatitis B virus, hepatitis C virus, and syphilis. The placenta is stored in -80°C, until a second seronegative result is obtained for HIV. Under a lamellar flow hood, the placenta is cleaned of any remaining blood clots with sterile Earle's solution (Life Technologies, Inc, Gaithersburg, MD) containing 50 ng/ml penicillin, 50 mg/ml streptomycin, 100 ng/ml neomycin, and 2.5 mg/ml amphothericin B. The amnion is separated from the rest of the chorion by blunt dissection *(Figure 3-1, left)*, and flattened on a 0.45 mm nitrocellulose filter paper, with the basement membrane surface up. Any residual blood is meticulously removed from the membrane. Sheets of the filter paper with the amniotic membrane are cut into pieces of 3x4 cm^2, and stored at -80°C in a medium containing equal volumes of Dulbeco's modified Eagle medium (DMEM, Life Technologies, Inc) and glycerol (Baxter Healthcare corporation, Stone Mountain, GA) until used for transplantation.

Pterygium Excision and Amniotic Membrane Transplantation *(Figure 3-2)*

All patients are anesthetized with a retrobulbar block. A lid-speculum is placed *(Figure 3-2.A)*. Several drops of 1:1000 epinephrine are applied topically in order to prevent excessive bleeding during extensive excision of the pterygium tissue *(Figure 3-2.B)*. Two 7-0 Vicryl traction sutures are placed episclerally 2 to 3 mm from the superior and inferior limbus, at 6 and 12 o'clock, to help mobilize the globe *(Figures 3-2.C, 3-2.D)*.

A pair of sharp Westcott Scissors was used to undermine the pterygium head along the limbal line *(Figure 3-2.E)*. After the scissors are well placed bellow the head, they are moved towards the cornea in a quick and decisive one-step movement as blunt dissection, until the head is completely separated from the cornea *(Figure 3-2.F)*. In cases of recurrent pterygium, a similar attempt of head dissection is made only if the corneal thickness in the area covered by the head appears normal. This is because the cornea may be thinner in this area due to previous surgical excisions.

The head is then grasped with a pointed 0.12 forceps, and the pterygium body is dissected along

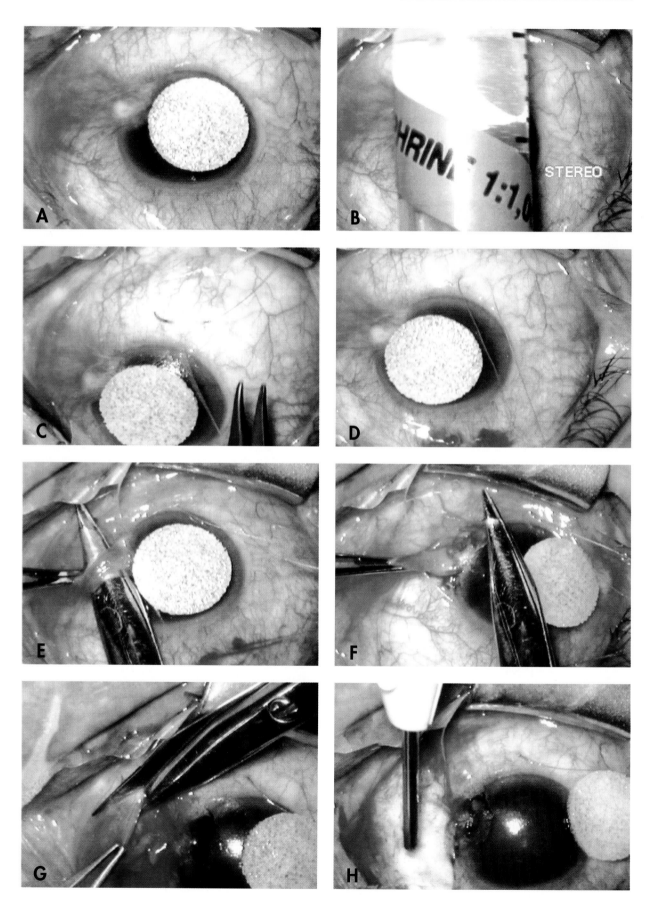

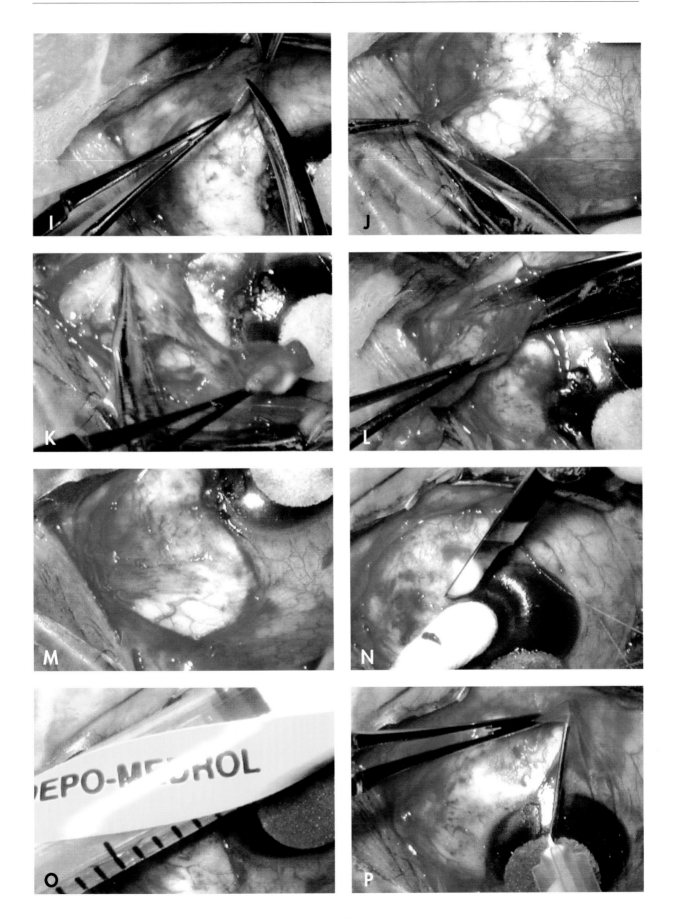

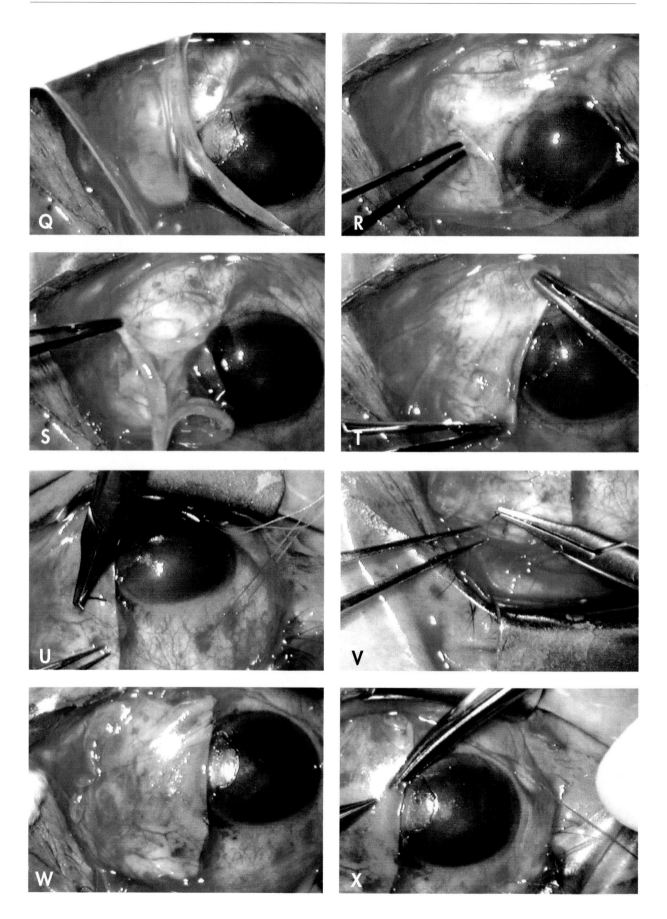

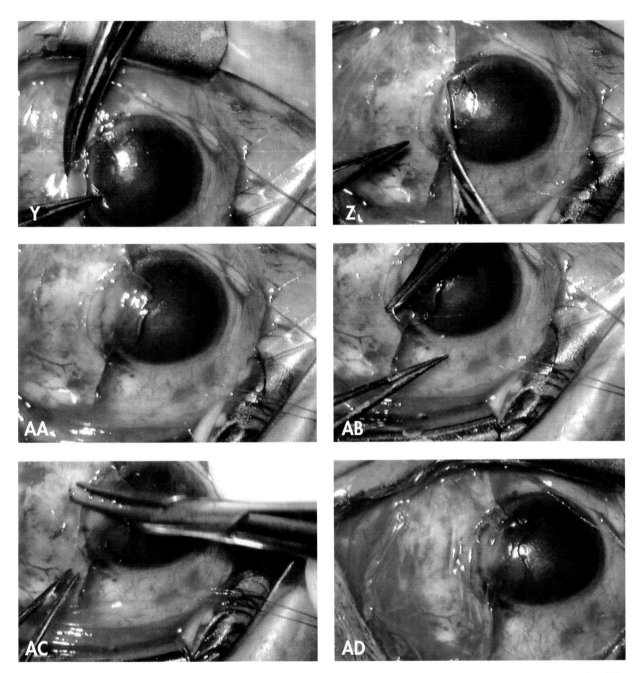

Figure 3-2. *Excision of a primary pterygium with a double-layered amniotic membrane transplantation. Retrobulbar anesthesia is used, and the lids are retracted with a speculum* **(A)**. *Epinephrine (1:1000) is applied topically to minimize bleeding* **(B)**. *Episcleral traction sutures are placed in the perilimbal area at 6 and 12 o'clock* **(C-D)**. *The pterygium head is undermined with a pair of sharp Westcott scissors* **(E)**, *followed by a blunt dissection of the head from the cornea* **(F)**. *The pterygium head and body are dissected off* **(G)**, *and cauterization is applied to control bleeding* **(H)**. *A radical removal of subconjunctival tissue is performed in the caruncle area and around the pterygium excision area, extending up to almost 180°* **(I-L)**. *Care is taken not to sever the medial rectal muscle fascia, which is revealed following this extensive tissue removal* **(M)**. *The corneal defect area is cleaned with a blade* **(N)**. *A corticosteroid is injected into the normal conjunctiva at the edge of excision* **(O-P)**. *The amniotic membrane is peeled off the carrier paper* **(Q)**, *and spread over the denuded scleral area, with the basement membrane side facing down* **(R)**. *The membrane is then folded so that the basement membrane side of its outer (superficial) layer is facing up (towards the surgeon)* **(S)**. *The folded edge of this double layered amniotic membrane is moved to cover the limbus* **(T)**, *and sutured with 10-0 nylon sutures to the episclera in the perilimbal area* **(U)**. *A continuous suture is used to secure the membrane nasally in the caruncle area* **(V-W)**. *In order to cover the corneal defect, a cut is made in the outer layer* **(X-Y)** *resulting in a pedicle flap that is spread with the basement membrane side facing down to cover the corneal defect as a patch* **(Z-AA)**. *The flap is secured with sutures to the cornea* **(AB-AC)**. *Final appearance* **(AD)**.

its upper and lower borders, separating it from the normal adjacent conjunctiva superiorly and inferiorly, and from the Tenon's capsule underneath *(Figure 3-2.G)*. This is completed by separating the body at the caruncle area. It must be noted that the true extent of the pterygium body is always larger than the area observed at the slit lamp. The true extent of the body may be close to 180°. Clues as to the extent of the body include distorted or convoluted episcleral vessels and a yellowish subconjuctival hue. In cases of a double-head pterygium, all of the inferior subconjunctival tissue may be involved, creating a continuous pterygial tissue. The removal will end up with defects extending nasal, temporal and inferior bulbar conjunctiva if pterygial tissue is to be removed in total.

Following removal of the body, a thorough and extensive removal of subconjunctival tissue is performed at the edges of the caruncle (in nasal pterygia). This tissue has no clearly defined borders. However it can be carefully dissected by holding its edge with a 0.12 forceps, and separating it from the adjacent conjunctiva and the underlying muscle's fascia or episclera *(Figures 3-2.I-3-2.L)*. C are must be taken not to severe the muscles fascia *(Figure 3-2.M)*. This is especially difficult in recurrent cases, where the fibrovascular tissue is adherent to the muscle. Cautery is performed to control bleeding *(Figure 3-2.H)*. The corneal defect area is polished with a blade and/or dental bur to remove any residual pterygial tissue from the excised head area *(Figure 3-2.N)*.

After completing the dissection of the subconjunctival tissue, a long-acting corticosteroid, triamcinolone acetonide (Kenalog), is injected via 27 gauge needle into the areas of normal conjunctiva adjacent to the border of the excised tissue *(Figures 3-2.O, 3-2.P)*.

In cases of a recurrent pterygium with symblepharon, the conjunctival epithelial tissue in the symblepharon area should be preserved and recessed to form the tarsal aspect of the fornix, and the subconjunctival fibrovascular tissue is similarly excised. After removal of the corneal portion of the pterygium, the conjunctiva is dissected from the underlying fibrovascular tissue. The subconjunctival tissue mass is dissected from the episclera and

removed. The freed conjunctival surface is then retracted down into the fornix. It may be advisable to assure fixation of the conjunctiva to the tarsal aspect of the lid by suturing the conjunctiva to the lid with two double-armed 5-0 black silk sutures. These sutures are tied externally to the skin with a small silicone tube.

After thawing the amniotic membrane is peeled from the carrier nitrocellulose paper under the microscope *(Figure 3-2.Q)*. It is spread over the denuded area to cover the bare sclera and the corneal defect *(Figure 3-2.R)*. The membrane should be applied so that the basement membrane side is facing upward. The way to distinguish the basement membrane surface from the stromal side of the membrane is by touching it with a sponge, i.e. Weckcel (Edward Weck & Company, Inc., Research Triangle Park, NC). The stromal side is sticky to, while the basement membrane side is not to the Weckcel's tip. The membrane is spread so that no wrinkle is seen. The edges of the membrane should be placed under the edges of the normal conjunctiva so that conjunctival epithelial cells may grow readily onto the amniotic membrane. Care should be taken to avoid bleeding trapped under the membrane, which may incite prolonged inflammation. The amniotic membrane is secured to the episclera with 10-0 nylon interrupted sutures perilimbally and to the cornea to allow a membrane flap to cover the corneal defect *(Figures 3-2.U, 3-2.V)*, and with 10-0 nylon continuous sutures to approximate the membrane to the caruncle area and to the conjunctival edge *(Figure 3-2.W)*.

At the end of surgery, the eye is patched with an antibiotic-corticosteroid ointment.

Surgical Modifications

In cases of a recurrent pterygium or large primary pterygium, the exposed rectal muscle is best protected with two layers of the amniotic membrane. The first layer should be placed on the rectus rectal muscle, with its basement membrane side down (facing the muscle). The second layer is placed above it, to cover the entire defect, with the basement membrane side up. The episcleral sutures will therefore include both membranes. This double layering may protect the rectal muscle from further adhesions and restriction.

An alternative to using two separate layers is to fold a bigger piece of the membrane in a way that the basement membrane sides face outside and the stromal sides face each other *(Figure 3-2.S)*. The membrane is placed over the defect, with the folded line near the limbus *(Figure 3-2.T)*. A small flap of the membrane can be cut in the limbus area *(Figures 3-2.X, 3-2.Y)*, and the flap can be retracted to cover the corneal defect *(Figures 3-2.Z, 3-2.AA)*. The flap is sutured to the cornea *(Figures 3-2.AB, 3-2.AC)*. This will ensure rapid epithelialization of the corneal defect with minimal or no scarring.

The amniotic membrane graft can be combined with a small conjunctival autograft (in the size of 2x8 mm) in a patient that had had previous pterygium surgeries with multiple recurrences, especially those with motility restriction. This conjunc-

tival graft is sutured over the amniotic membrane graft in an orientation parallel to the limbus. The incorporation of a conjunctival autograft can facilitate a faster epithelialization of the membrane graft, which is crucial to prevent recurrence.

Post-operative Management

At the first post-operative day, most patients would feel comfortable with almost no pain. Pain is frequently noted in pterygium surgeries when the corneal defect and some of the episcleral area are left uncovered. The amniotic membrane graft is usually completely epithelialized by the end of the second to third week *(Figure 3-3)*, when the sutures are removed. Normally, patients are treated with topical corticosteroid for a period of 4-8 weeks. When areas of marked fibrovascular proliferation, or congested conjunctival vessels are noted, espe-

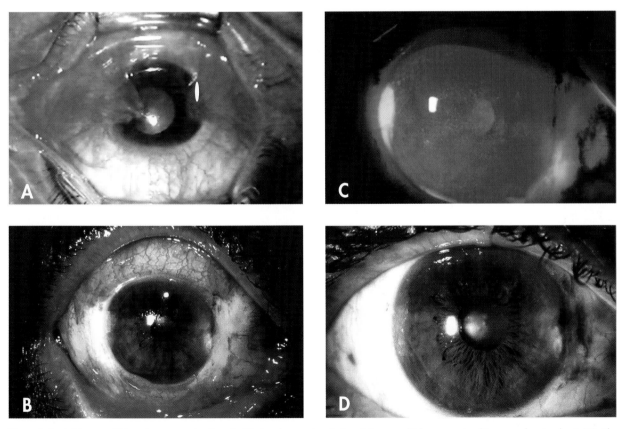

Figure 3-3. *A 74 year-old female presented with a double-head pterygium in her right eye, which was encroaching onto the visual axis* **(A)**. *She complained of irritation and redness. The double head pterygial tissues were removed to include the inferior bulbar conjunctiva. The resulting conjunctival defect was covered with an amniotic membrane graft. Two weeks following surgery her eye was quiet with complete epithelialization of the membrane graft* **(B-C)**. *At 15 months postoperatively she has a grade 1 appearance (also see Fig. 3-4) with a good cosmetic outcome* **(D)**.

cially at the host conjunctiva near the excision, local injections of triamcinolone acetonide (Kenalog) are administered. When a pyogenic granuloma develops, it is treated by excision if it is pedunculated, or with triamcinolone injection if it has a broad base.

POST-OPERATIVE OUTCOME

The final outcome is evaluated using a grading system on a scale of 1 to 4, as previously described *(Figure 3-4)*.[6] Grade 1 indicates a normal appearance of the operated site. Grade 2 indicates indicated fine episcleral vessels in the excised area, extending to the limbus, without any fibrous tissue. Grade 3 demonstrates fibrovascular tissue in the excised area, reaching to the limbus, but not invading the cornea. Grade 4 represents a true recurrence, with fibrovascular tissue invading the cornea.

We have previously compared amniotic mem-

brane transplantation for pterygium surgery with two other methods: conjunctival autograft and primary closure.[6] In the amniotic membrane group, the true recurrence rate (grade 4) was 10.9% and 37.5% for primary and recurrent pterygia, respectively. The conjunctival autograft group had recurrence rates of 2.6% and 9.1% for primary and recurrent pterygia, respectively, while the primary closure group had a 45% recurrence for primary pterygia. It should be noted that recurrence for amniotic membrane group tends to be delayed as compared to primary closure, suggesting that there is an ongoing process to activate recurrence.

In a more recent study, we have demonstrated that a further reduction of the recurrence rate can be achieved by amniotic membrane transplantation for pterygium surgery (Solomon and Tseng, manuscript submitted). In a prospective study of 54 eyes of 54 patients, we noted that the true recurrence rate was 3.0% for primary and 9.5% for recurrent pterygia, respectively, after a mean follow-up of 12.3 ± 4.4

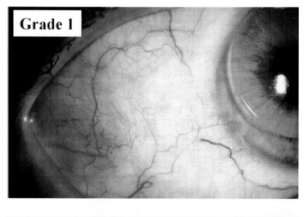
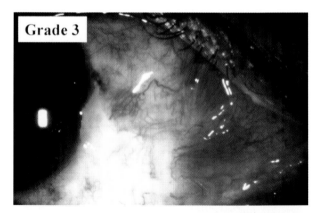
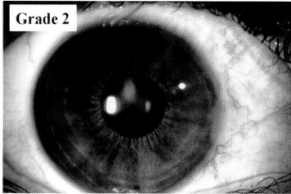
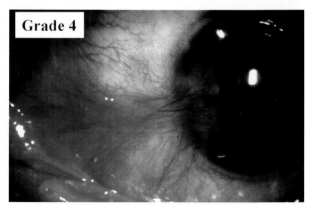

Figure 3-4. *Outcome grading following pteryium surgery.* **Grade 1** *- a normal appearance of the operated site.* **Grade 2** *- fine episcleral vessels in the excised area.* **Grade 3** *- fibrovascular tissue in the excised area, reaching to the limbus, but not invading the cornea.* **Grade 4** *- fibrovascular tissue invading the cornea (i.e., true recurrence).*

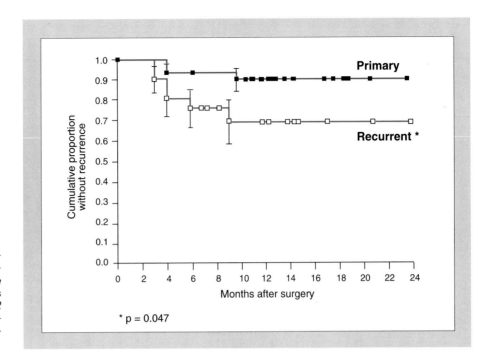

Figure 3-5. *Kaplan-Meyer survival curves of primary and recurrent pterygia. The cumulative incidence of recurrence-free eyes (i.e., grades 1 and 2) at 12 months was 0.90 ± 0.06 for primary and 0.69 ± 0.11 for recurrent pterygia.*

months (range 6.1 - 22.9 months). Survival analysis showed that the cumulative proportion of recurrence free eyes (grades 1 and 2) at 12 months was 0.90 ± 0.06 for primary pterygia compared to 0.69 ± 0.11 for recurrent pterygia *(Figure 3-5)* (p=0.047).

Out of these 54 eyes, 11 eyes had a double-head primary pterygium (an example is seen in Figure 3-3). Ten of these 11 eyes (90.9%) ended up with a grade 1 or 2 postoperative appearance, while only one eye had a true recurrence.

Therefore, the outcome in double-head pterygia was similar to that of single-head one. We attribute this success to the extensive tissue removal to include that from the inferior fornix.

The complications encountered included pyogenic granuloma in 5 eyes, two cases of symblepharon formation, and one case of motility restriction. Postoperatively, subconjunctival injections of Kenalog were given to 17 eyes, within the first 3 months, when areas of increased fibrovascular activity were noted in the operated area. Of these cases, five eventually progressed to either grade 3 or grade 4 appearance. In two of the eyes injected with Kenalog, a transient increase of the intraocular pressure was noted.

CONCLUSIONS

Our experience with amniotic membrane grafts for pterygium surgery show that this technique is useful for both primary and recurrent pterygia, in achieving a low recurrence rate, quick rehabilitation of the conjunctival surface, low incidence of complications, and an agreeable cosmetic result.

This is accomplished through a physiologic reconstruction of the excision area, using a human-derived basement membrane, which serves as a carrier for growth of a healthy epithelium, as well as an agent that prevents scarring and inflammation. Its main advantage is in the ability to restore large excised areas, e.g., in double-head or large recurrent pterygia, where a conjunctival autograft is not possible, or in cases where the conjunctiva is already scarred from previous surgery, or has to be reserved for a possible glaucoma-filtering surgery.

Further modifications of our method, such as combination with a conjunctival autograft or with intraoperative application of mitomycin C, can be tailored to individual cases.

References

1. Trelford JD, Trelford-Sauder M. The amnion in surgery, past and present. *Am J Obstet Gynecol.* 1979; 134:833-845.

2. de Rotth A. Plastic repair of conjunctival defects with fetal membrane. *Arch Ophthalmol.* 1940;23:522-525.

3. Sorsby A, Symons HM. Amniotic membrane grafts in caustic burns of the eye. *Br J Ophthalmol.* 1946; 30:337-345.

4. Sorsby A, Haythorne J, Reed H. Further experience with amniotic membrane grafts in caustic burns of the eye. *Br J Ophthalmol.* 1947;31:409-418.

5. Kim JC, Tseng SCG. Transplantation of preserved human amniotic membrane for surface reconstruction in severely damaged rabbit corneas. *Cornea.* 1995; 14:473-484.

6. Prabhasawat P, Barton K, Burkett G, Tseng SCG. Comparison of conjunctival autografts, amniotic membrane grafts and primary closure for pterygium excision. *Ophthalmology.* 1997;104:974-985.

7. Shimazaki J, Shinozaki N, Tsubota K. Transplantation of amniotic membrane and limbal autograft for patients with recurrent pterygium associated with symblepharon. *Br J Ophthalmol.* 1998;82:235-240.

8. Tseng SCG, Prabhasawat P, Lee S-H. Amniotic membrane transplantation for conjunctival surface reconstruction. *Am J Ophthalmol.* 1997;124:765-774.

9. Franch A, Rama P, Lambiase A, Ponzin D, Caprioglio G. Human amniotic membrane transplantation. *Invest. Ophthalmol. Vis. Sci.* 39, S90. 1998. Ref Type: Abstract

10. Terranova VP, Lyall RM. Chemotaxis of human gingival epithelial cells to laminin. A mechanism for epithelial cell apical migration. *J Periodontol.* 1986; 57:311-317.

11. Khodadoust AA, Silverstein AM, Kenyon KR, Dowling JE. Adhesion of regenerating corneal epithelium. The role of basement membrane. *Am J Ophthalmol.* 1968; 65:339-348.

12. Sonnenberg A, Calafat J, Janssen H, Daams H, van der Raaij-Helmer LMH, Falcinoi R, Kennel S, Aplin JD, Baker J, Loizidou M, Garrod D. Integrin a6/b4 complex is located in hemidesmosomes, suggesting a major role in epidermal cell-basement membrane adhesion. *J Cell Biol.* 1991;113:907-917.

13. Guo M, Grinnell F. Basement membrane and human epidermal differentiation in vitro. *J Invest Dermatol.* 1989;93:372-378.

14. Streuli CH, Bailey N, Bissell MJ. Control of mammary epithelial differentiation: basement membrane induces tissue-specific gene expression in the absence of cell-cell interaction and morphological polarity. *J Cell Biol.* 1991;115:1383-1395.

15. Kurpakus MA, Stock EL, Jones JCR. The role of the basement membrane in differential expression of keratin proteins in epithelial cells. *Dev Biol.* 1992;150:243-255.

16. Barcellos-Hoff MH, Aggeler J, Ram TG, Bissell MJ. Functional differentiation and alveolar morphogenesis of primary mammary cultures on reconstituted basement membrane. *Development.* 1989;105:223-235.

17. Boudreau N, Sympson CJ, Werb Z, Bissell MJ. Suppression of ICE and apoptosis in mammary epithelial cells by extracellular matrix. *Science.* 1995;267:891-893.

18. Boudreau N, Werb Z, Bissell MJ. Suppression of apoptosis by basement membrane requires three-dimensional tissue organization and withdrawal from the cell cycle. *Proc Natl Acad Sci USA.* 1996;93:3500-3513.

19. Lee S-H, Tseng SCG. Amniotic membrane transplantation for persistent epithelial defects with ulceration. *Am J Ophthalmol.* 1997;123:303-312.

20. Taylor RJ, Wang MX. Rate of re-epithelialization following amniotic membrane transplantation. *Invest. Ophthalmol. Vis. Sci.* 39, S1038. 1998.

21. Azuara-Blanco A, Pillai CT, Sarhan A, Dua HS. Amniotic membrane transplantation for ocular surface reconstruction. *Invest. Ophthalmol. Vis. Sci.* 39, S428. 1998.

22. Cho B, Djalilian AR, Obritsch WF, Mattteson DM, Chan CC, Holland EJ. Conjunctival epithelial cells cultured on human amniotic membrane do not transdifferentiate into corneal epithelial type cells. *Invest. Ophthalmol. Vis. Sci.* 39, S428. 1998.

23. Meller D, Tseng SCG. Conjunctival epithelial differentiation on amniotic membrane. *Invest Ophthalmol Vis Sci.* 1999;40:878-886.

24. Prabhasawat P, Tseng SCG. Impression cytology study of epithelial phenotype of ocular surface reconstructed by preserved human amniotic membrane. *Arch Ophthalmol.* 1997;115:1360-1367.

25. Tseng SCG, Li D-Q, Ma X. Suppression of TGF- b1, b2, b3, and TGF-b receptor II expression and myofibroblast differentiation in human corneal and limbal fibroblasts by amniotic membrane matrix. *J Cell Physiol.* 1999; 179:325-335.

26. Wang MX, Gray T, Prabhasawat P, Ma X, Ding F-Y, Hernandez E, Sana, Sanabria O, Culbertson WW, Hanna K, Forster RK, Tseng SCG. Corneal haze is reduced by amniotic membrane matrix in excimer laser photoablation in rabbits. *Invest Ophthalmol Vis Sci.* 1997; 38:405S.

27. Kim JS, Park SW, Kim JH, Lee SI, Yang HN, Kim JC. Temporary amniotic membrane graft promotes healing and inhibits protease activity in corneal wound induced by alkali burns in rabbits. *Invest. Ophthalmol. Vis. Sci.* 39, S90. 1998.

28. Sato H, Shimazaki J, Shinozaki K, Tsubota K. Role of growth factors for ocular surface reconstruction after amniotic membrane transplantation. *Invest. Ophthalmol. Vis. Sci.* 39, S428. 1998.

29. Park WC, Tseng SCG. Temperature cooling reduces keratocyte death in excimer laser ablated corneal and skin wounds. *Invest. Ophthalmol. Vis. Sci.* 39, S449. 1998.

30. Na BK, Hwang JH, Shin EJ, Song CY, Jeong JM, Kim JC. Analysis of human amniotic membrane components as proteinase inhibitors for development of therapeutic agent of recalcitrant keratitis. *Invest. Ophthalmol. Vis. Sci.* 39, S90. 1998.

31. Kim JC, Tseng SCG. The effects on inhibition of corneal neovascularization after human amniotic membrane transplantation in severely damaged rabbit corneas. *Korean J Ophthalmol.* 1995;9:32-46.

32. Tsubota K, Satake Y, Ohyama M, Toda I, Takano Y, Ono M, Shinozaki N, Shimazaki J. Surgical reconstruction of the ocular surface in advanced ocular cicatricial pemphigoid and Stevens-Johnson syndrome. *Am J Ophthalmol.* 1996;122:38-52.

33. Shimazaki J, Yang H-Y, Tsubota K. Amniotic membrane transplantation for ocular surface reconstruction in patients with chemical and thermal burns. *Ophthalmology.* 1997;104:2068-2076.

34. Tseng SCG, Prabhasawat P, Barton K, Gray T, Meller D. Amniotic membrane transplantation with or without limbal allografts for corneal surface reconstruction in patients with limbal stem cell deficiency. *Arch Ophthalmol.* 1998;116:431-441.

35. Choi YS, Kim JY, Wee WR, Lee JH. Effect of the application of human amniotic membrane on rabbit corneal wound healing after excimer laser photorefractive keratectomy. *Cornea.* 1998;17:389-395.

36. Solomon A, Li D-Q, Lee S-B, Tseng SCG. Differential regulation of Collagenase (MMP-1), Stromelysin (MMP-3) and uokinase-type Plasminogen-Activator (uPA) in cultured human conjunctival and primary pterygium body fibroblasts by inflammatory cytokines. *Invest Ophthalmol Vis Sci* 2000;41 (in press).

4

ANTIPROLIFERATIVE THERAPY FOR PTERYGIUM SURGERY

Joseph Frucht-Pery, M.D. — Charalambos S. Siganos, M.D.

Pterygia are a common problem in many parts of the world. Pterygium manifestations include hyperemia, tearing and symptoms such as burning, foreign body and itching sensations. In some cases, chronic or intermittent inflammatory events require medical treatment and may significantly interfere with the normal style of life of an individual. Furthermore invasion of pterygium tissue into the cornea may induced marked corneal astigmatism. In extreme cases, growth of vascular tissue into the visual axis may severely affect the visual function and even cause legal blindness.

Surgery is the only method available to remove pterygium from the cornea. The indications for a surgical procedure include a progression of the neovascular tissue towards the visual axis and induced astigmatism. However, in many patients the discomfort and the cosmetic appearance of constantly irritated red eyes becomes an indication for surgical intervention. Unfortunately, excision of the pterygium is not effective in all patients. According to the ophthalmic literature, the rate of recurrent growth of fibrovascular tissue onto the cornea after primary pterygium excision surgery ranges from 2% to 89%. The different in the post-operative outcome is not well understood and is caused by the different selection criteria of the patients for surgery, by the efficacy of the various surgical procedures and the adjunctive intraoperative and postoperative treatments. At the present time, there are no

simple answers, nor is there a broad consensus of the experts as to the optimal approach to the treatment of pterygia.

The fact that after pterygium surgery, the fibrovascular tissue proliferates rapidly in one case but not in another suggests that individual factors of wound healing may be of critical importance. Therefore, many attempts have been made over past decades to control or arrest the post-operative proliferation of fibrovascular tissue.

Beta irradiation and medications such as thiotepa and Mitomycin C have been used to control tissue proliferation.

THIOTEPA

Thiotepa (triethylene thiophosphoramide) is an alkalating agent, an analogue of nitrogen mustard. It inhibits the division and mitosis of cells in rapidly proliferating tissue.[1]

Thiotepa was first published in 1962 as an adjunctive treatment after pterygium excision.[2] A 0.05% solution of thiotepa was used for 6-8 weeks.[3]

Kleis and Pleo found 8.3% recurrence rate of pterygium in the thiotepa-treated group as compared with 31.3% in the control eyes.[4]

Several complications have been reported including conjunctival injection, allergic reactions, poliosis, black pigment deposits, headache, photo-phobia, irritation, foreign body sensation, scleral perforation and pseudomonas aeruginosa-induced sclerokeratitis with poor vision outcome.[5-8]

However, the most devastating complication was the skin pigmentation on the eyelids and around the eyes which was induced by sunlight exposure after thiotepa application[2] and was the reason for the discontinuation of thiotepa use by most ophthalmologists.

BETA-RADIATION

Beta-radiation is induced by Strontium 90. Beta-radiation inhibits the mitosis of rapidly dividing cells and is capable of arresting the proliferation of fibrovascular tissue.[9]

Strontium 90 application was used after excision of pterygia. A total dose of 1200 rads to 6000 rads was applied as a single application within the first 24 hours after surgery or in divided doses over a period of six weeks.[10-18, 23]

The recurrence rate of pterygium after surgical excision and adjunctive application of beta-radiation varied from 0.5% to 33%: mostly less than 13%.[11-22] MacKemzie et al. followed their patients for a period of ten years and reported 12% recurrence rate. However, only 50% [585 patients] of the treated patients were available for follow-up.[15]

We have used beta-radiation for more than 15 years and thought that the treatment was very efficacious. It is therefore surprising to discover a 20% recurrence rate of pterygium in a small group of patients who were randomly treated with beta-radiation and served as controls for Mitomycin C groups.[23]

The adverse effects of the beta radiation include mild complications such as mild conjunctivitis, symblepharon, iris atrophy, infections, scleral ulcerations and necrosis and loss of sight.[10, 14-16, 24-27] MacKenzie et al discovered a 13% rate of scleromalacia in a ten-year follow-up study.[15] More importantly, 4.5% of these cases had severe scleromalacia which occurred many years after the application of beta radiation. Scleral thinning was associated (but not significant) with a greater dose of beta-radiation.[15] Severe microbial endophthalmitis

including fungal and pseudomonas infections was reported after application of beta radiation and led to an eye enucleation in one case.[10,15,26-27] It appears that formation of plaques at the sight of scleral necrosis may harbor micro-organisms and predispose the patient to severe infections.[29] Auto-transplantation of conjunctiva could be one solution in cases with scleral necrosis and in cases of plaque formation.

At the present time, beta-irradiation is being used by ophthalmologists all over the world. However, patients and ophthalmologists should be aware of the life-long risks of these complications and patients should be followed-up by ophthalmologists for many years after receiving beta-radiation.

MITOMYCIN C

Mitomycin C (MMC) is an antibiotic-antineoplastic agent that selectively inhibits the synethesis of DNA, cellular RNA and protein, and has a long-term effect on cellular proliferation.[28,29] MMC use is limited to bladder tumors and nonresponsive adenocarcinomas because of its toxicity to blood stem cells and other organs.

Kunimoto and Mori used MMC in pterygium surgery in 1963 but appearance of complications restricyted the use of the drug.[30] Singh et al. applied drops of MMC at concentrations of 0.1% or 0.04% four times daily for two weeks.[31] Although the recurrence rate of pterygium after MMC use was only 2.3% (and 89% in controls), 0.1% MMC drops caused ocular pain, tearing, superficial punctate keratopathy, iritis, conjunctival irritation and delay of conjunctival wound healing. On the other hand 0.4% MMC had fewer complications.[31] Hayasaka found a comparable rate of recurrence of pterygium when 0.04% mitomycin (tid/one week) or 0.02% mitomycin (bid/ five days) were used. However, MMC 0.04% presented more complications including scleral ulceration.[32] MMC 0.02% was also efficacious in patients with recurrent pterygium (5% recurrence rate).[33] Many authors including us, reported less than 10% pterygium recurrence rates using MMC 0.02%, bid for 5 days.[23,7,34-38]

Despite of the low pterygium recurrence rates, ophthalmic society all over the world became concerned with the uncontrolled use of topical MMC drops at home which caused severe ocular complications. Ocular pain, photophobia, iritis, avascularity of the limbal areas, scleral melting and scleral or corneal perforations have been reported.[31,32-34,39-50]

Rubinfeld[40] reported a group of patients with incapacitating photophobia, pain scleral melting, corneal edema, melting and perforation, iritis and corectopia, secondary glaucoma and cataract formation. Some of these patients had immune disorders such as rosacea, keratitis sicca and ichtiosis: they used drops of MMC 0.04% for a period longer than 2 weeks and did not show-up for follow-up.[40] It appears that appropriate selection criteria are critical for the prevention of severe complications. Patients with immune disorders, dry eyes, ocular surface disorders and with possible compliance problems should not be treated with topical MMC drops at home.

The increasing experience of MMC use in glaucoma surgery and the significant inhibitory effect on tenon fibroblast proliferation in the bleb by a single intraoperative application of MMC, convinced us to try an intraoperative, single use of topical MMC for pterygium surgery.

My surgical technique was designed for an 'intraoperative, single use of MMC approach for pterygium surgery' *(Figure 4-1)*. The procedure starts with a wide dissection of conjunctiva from the underlying from the underlying pterygium. In extreme cases the dissection may proceed above the muscle toward the caruacula. In order to preserve most of the conjunctival tissue the dissected conjunctiva is separated from the head of pterygium at the limbus. Thereafter, the pterygium head is dissected from the cornea and the whole pterygium tissue is excised, excluding the conjunctiva. A sponge soaked with MMC 0.02% is placed on the bare sclera and the conjunctiva is pulled over the sponge like a blanket. The sponge is kept under the conjunctiva for five, in order to inhibit the activity of the remaining tenon capsule fibroblasts and pterygium fibroblasts. The application of the MMC under the conjunctiva decreased the exposure of the conjunctival epithelial cells to the drug and did not

affect the rapid proliferation of these cells in order to cover the non-epithelialized wound after the surgery.[45-46] After removal of the sponge, the ocular surface is rinsed with 30 ml of BSS: Thereafter, the conjunctiva is tightly sutured to the sclera with 10-nylon stitches, leaving 1 to 2 mm of bare sclera. No cauterization is used (or required) because the pressure of the sponge and the affect of MMC on endothelial vascular cells led to the formation of non-bleeding ocular surface. On the other hand, excessive cauterization may cause an extra inflammatory response and a delay of wound healing, which may be critical after MMC use. We found that single dose intraoperative application of MMC 0.02% for 5 minutes had only 5% of post-operative recurrence of pterygium (47% recurrence in untreated controls).[45-46]

Many authors adjusted this technique. Intraoperative single doses of MMC of 0.01% to 0.04% were used for 3 to 5 minutes with excellent results of 3.3% to 12.5% of recurrence rate of pterygium.[48-50]

The ideal time span of the single MMC dose exposure during the pterygium surgery is not yet determined. Lann et al.[51] found that five rates of 8%, as compared to 22.9% and 42.9% after use of the same concentrations for three minutes only. We used 5 minutes exposure for several years, however, nowadays we use 3 minutes exposure time and our recurrence rates of pterygium remains at a level of 6.0% [unpublished data]. Although we feel that the time of exposure is very important and should properly be studied in the future, the correct placement of the MMC-sponge under the conjunctiva is as well extremely important and should be executed precisely. We agree that in recurrent pterygia or in very fleshy and progressive cases longer period of exposure might be of a greater benefit.

Single intraoperative use of MMC is relatively safe and some authors found the surgery uncomplicated.[46,49,53] Other complications included temporary delayed conjunctival wound healing[47,50] conjunctival granulomas[47] and chemosis on the first post-operative day.[54] No late complications post-single intraoperative MMC-use were reported except for one case reported of corneal melting.[55]

Although the optimal dosage (concentration or

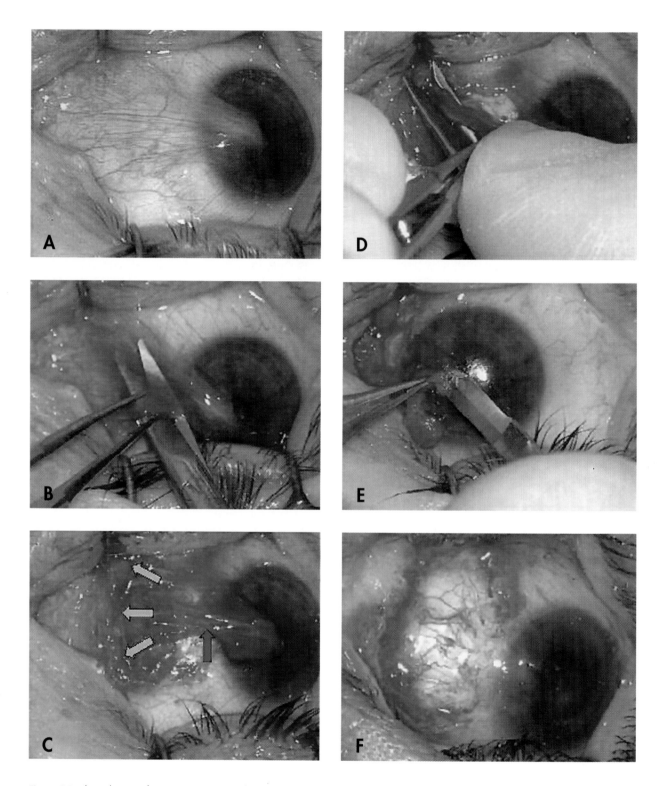

Figure 4-1. *The technique of pterygium excision with intraoperative mitomycin use.*
A. *Large vascularized pterygium.*
B. *Dissection of the conjunctiva from the body of the pterygium.*
C. *Exposed body of pterygium [dark arrow]. The conjunctiva is contacted in the nasal side [white arrows].*
D. *Excision of the nasal aspect of the pterygium.*
E. *Dissection of the head of pterygium.*
F. *Bare sclera.*

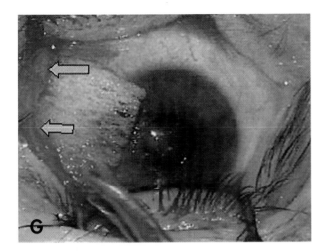

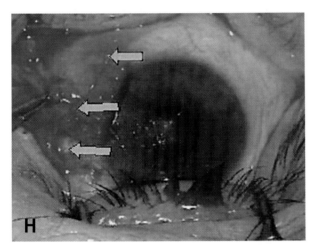

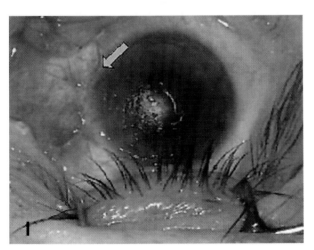

Figure 4-1 (continued). *The technique of pterygium excision with intraoperative mitomycin use.*
G. *Placing the MMC soaked sponge under the conjunctiva (arrows).*
H. *Pulling the conjunctiva with forceps over the sponge for 3 to 5 minutes. (Arrows indicate the edge of the conjunctiva).*
I. *Suturing the conjunctiva to the sclera leaving 1 to 2 mm of bare sclera. (Arrow indicates the edge of the conjunctiva).*

duration) of intraoperative application of MMC has not yet been determined, studies indicate that a single dose intraoperative use is as effective as post-operative use of the MMC drops at home. Cardilo et al.[52] reported similar pterygium recurrence rates (4.0% to 6.6%) after application of intraoperative MMC (0.02% or 0.04%) or post-operative drops of MMC (0.02% or 0.04%).

While the ophthalmologist has reasonable control when MMC is applied intraoperatively, use of MMC at home is compliance-dependent, costly and is controlled by the patient. Most ophthalmologists who use MMC will prefer intraoperative rather than post-operative application of MMC. Patient selection has to be very careful, and patients should be instructed to continue with periodical examinations for many years to come.

REFERENCES

1. Olander K, Halk KG, Halk GM. Management of ptery-gia: should thiotepa be used? *Ann Ophthalmol* 1978; 10(7): 853-862.

2. Jaros PA, DeLuise VP, Pingueculae and pterygia. S*rv Ophthalmol* 1974; 6:739.

3. Ehrlich D. The management of pterygium. *Ophthalmic Surg* 1977; 8(2): 23-30.

4. Kleis W, Pico G. Thiotepa therapy to prevent postoperative pterygium occurrence and neovascularization. *Am J Ophthalmol* 1973; 76(3): 371-373.

5. Harben DJ, Cooper PH, Rodman OG. Thiotepa-induced leukodema. *Arch Dermatol* 1979; 115 (8): 973-974.

6. Arsegadoo ER. Thio-tepa, and corticosteroid in the treatment of pterygium. *Am J Ophthalmol* 1972; 74(5): 960-963.

7. Ngoy D, Kayembe L. A comperative study of thio-tepa and mitomycin C in the treatment of pterygium. Preliminary results. *J Fr Ophthalmol* 1998; 21(2):96-102.

8. Farrell PL, Smith RE. Bacterial Corneoscleritis complicating pterygium excision. *Am J Ophthalmol* 1989 May 15; 107(5): 515-7.

9. Adamis AP, Stark T, Kenyon KR. The management of pterygium. *Ophthalmol Clin North Am* 1990; 3:611.

10. Tarr KH, Constable IJ. Late complications of pterygium tretament. *Br J Ophthalmol* 1980 Jul; 64(7): 498-505.

11. Alaniz-Camino F. The use of postoperative beta radiation in the treatment of pterygia. *Ophthalmic Surg* 1982 Dec; 13(12); 1022-1025.

12. Aswad ML, Baum J. Optimal Tratment for postoperative irradiation of pterygia. *Ophthalmology* 1987 Nov; 94(11): 1450-1451.

13. Campbell OR, Amendola BE, Brady LW. Recurrement pterygia: resulats of postoperative tratment with Sr-90 applications. *Radiology* 1990 Feb; 1974 (2):565-566.

14. Beyer DC. Pterygia: single-fraction postoperative beta irradiation. *Radiology* 1991 Feb.178(2),569-571.

15. MacKenzie FD, Hirst LW, Kynaston B, Bain C. Recurrence rate and complications after beta irradiation for pterygia. *Ophthalmology* 1991 Dec;98(12):1778-1780.

16. Dusenbery KE, Alul IH, Holland EJ, Khan FM, Levitt SH. Beta irradiation of recurrent pterygia: results and complications. *Int J Radiat Oncol Biol Phys* 1992;24(2) -315-320.

17. Wilder RB, Buatti JM, ShImm DS, Harari PM, Rogoff EE, Cassady JR. Pterygium treated with excision and postoperative beta irradiation. *Int J Radiat Oncol Biol Phys* 1992,23(3).533-537.

18. Paryani SB, Scott WP, Wells JW, Johnson DW, Chobe RJ, Kuruvilla A, Schoeppel S, Deshmukh A. Management of pterygium with surgery and radiation therapy. The north Florida Pterygium Study Group. *Int J Radiat Oncol Biol Phys* 1994 Jan 1;28(1):101-103.

19. Neal AJ, Irwin C, Hope-Stone HF. The role of strontium-90 beta irradiation in the management of pterygium. *Clin Oncol* (R Coll Radiol) 1991 Mar; 3(2): 105-109.

20. Cooper JS. Postoperative irradiation of pterygia: ten more years of experience. *Radiology* 1978 Sep; 128 (3):753-756.

21. Halk GM, Ellis GS, Nowell JF. The management of pterygia with special reference to surgery combined with beta irradiation. *Trans Am Acad Ophthalmol Otolaryngol* 1962;66;776-84

22. King JH Jr. The pterygium: brief reviw and evaluation of certain methods of treatment. Arch Ophthalmol 1950:44;854-69.

23. Fricht-PeryJ, Ilsar M. The use of low-dose mitomycin C for prevention of recurrent pterygium. *Ophthalmology* 1994;101(4):759-762.

24. Tarr KH, Constable IJ. Pseudomonas endophthalmitis associated with scleral necrosis. *Br J Ophthalmol* 1980 Sep:64(9): 515-517.

25. Farrell PL, Smith RE. Bacterial Corneoscleritiscomplicating pterygium excision. *Am J Ophthalmol* 1989 May 15;107(5):515-517.

26. Moriarty AP, Crwford GJ, McAllister IL, Constable IJ. Fungal corneoscleritis complicating beta-irradiation-induced scleral necrosis following pterygium excision. *Eye* 1993;7 (Pt4): 525-528.

27. Morirty AP, Crawford GJ, McAllister IL, Constable IJ. Severe coneoscleral infection. A complication of beta irradiation scleral necrosis following pterygium excision. *Arch Ophthalmol* 1993 Jul;111(7):947-951.

28. Gilman AG, Rall TW, Niles AS, Taylor P, eds. Goodman and Gilman's. *The pharmacological basis of theurapeutics*, 8th ed. New York: Pergamon Press, 1990; 1247-1248.

29. Bowman WC, Rand MJ, eds. Textbook of pharmacology 2nd ed., Blackwell, Oxford, 1980;3:14-5.

30. Kunimoto N, Mori S. Studies on the pterygium. Part IV. A treatment for pterygium. *Ophthalmology* 1988 15;106(6):715-718.

33. Hayasaka S, Noda S, Yamamoto Y, Sgtogawa T. Postoperative instillation of mitomycin C in the treatment of recurrent pterygium. *Ophthalmic Surg* 1989;20:715-718.

34. Chayakul V. Postoperative mitomycin-C eue drop and beta radiation in the treatment of pterygia. *J Med Assoc thai* 1991;74(9):373-376.

35. Moller DE, Goder GJ. Local mitomycin C therapy after excision of pterygium. *Klin Monatsbl Augenheilkd* 1992;200(3):231-232.

36. Simona F, Anastasi-Forni C, Benedetti C, Failla FG, Rossi FM, Meyer U. Adjuvant treatment with mitomicyn eyedrops after pterygium excision: Ticino experience. *Klin Monatsbl Augenheilkd* 1994;204(5):409-412.

37. Rachmiel R., Leiba H., Levartovsky S., Results of treatment with topical mitomycin C 0.02% following excision of primari pterygium. *Br J Ophthalmol* 1995; 79 (3): 233-6.

38. Mahar PS. Conjunctival autograft versus topical mitomycin C in treatment of pterygium. *Eye* 1997; 11: 790-792.54. Demirok A., Simsek S., Cinal A., Yasar T. Intraoperative application of mitomycin C in the surgical treatment of pterygium. *Eur J Ophthalmol* 1998; 8 (3) : 153-156.

39. Ngoy D., Kayembe L. A comparative study of thio-tepa and mitomycin C in the treatment of pterygium. Preliminary results. *J Fr Ophthalmol* 1998; 21 (2): 96-102.

40. Rubinfeld RS, Pfister RR, Stein RM, Foster CS, Martin NF, Stoleiu S., Talley AR, Speaker MG. Serious complications of topical mitomycin C after pterygium surgery. *Ophthalmology* 1992; 9 (11): 1647-154.

41. Ewing-Chow DA, Romanchuk KG, Gilmour GR, Underhill JH, Olimenhaga DB. Corneal melting after pterygium removal followed by topical mitomycin C therapy. *Can J Ophthalmol* 1992; 27 (4): 197-199.

42. Dunn JP, Seamone CD, Ostler HB, Nickel BL, Beallo A. Development of scleral ulceration and calcification after pterygium excision and mitomycin therapy. *Am J Ophthalmol* 1991 15; 112 (3): 343-344.

43. A. Fujitani, S. Hayasaka, Y. Shibuya, S. Noda. Corneoscleral ulceration and corneal perforation after pterygium excision and topical Mitomycin C treatment. *Ophthalmologica* 1993; 207: 162-4.

44. S. Gupta, S. Basti. Corneoscleral ciliary body and vitreoretinal toxicity after excessive instilation of mitomycin C. *Am J Ophthalmol* 1992; 114: 1503-4.

45. Frucht-Pery J., Ilsar M., Hemo I. Single dosage of mitomycin C for prevention of recurrent pterygium: preliminary report. *Cornea* 1994; 13 (5): 411-413.

46. Frucht-Pery J., Siganos CS, Ilsar M. Intraoperative application of topical mitomycin C for pterygium surgery. *Ophthalmology* 1996; 103 (4):674-647.

47. Cano-Parra J., Diaz-Liopis M., Maldonado MJ, Vila E., Menezo JL. Prospective trial of intraoperative mitomycin C in the treatment of primary pterygium. *Br J Ophthalmol* 1995; 79 (5): 439-441.

48. Mastropasqua L., Capineto P., Ciancaglini M., Gallenga PE. Long term results of intraoperative mitomycin C in the treatment of recurrent pterygium. *Br J Ophthalmol* 1966; 80: 288-291.

49. Manning CA, Kloess PM, Diaz MD, Yee RW. Intraoperative mitomycin in primary pterygium excision. A prospective randomised trial. *Ophthalmol.* 1997; 104: 844-848.

50. Helal M., Messiha N., Amaiem A. et al. Intraoperative mitomycin C versus postoperatve mitomycin C for the treatment of pterygium. *Ophthalmic Surg. and Lasers* 1996; 27: 674-678.

51. Lam DS, Wong AK, Fan DS, Chew S. Kwok PS, Tso MO. Intraoperative mitomycin C to prevent recurrence of pterygium after excision: a 30-month follow-up study. *Ophthalmology* 1998; 105 (5): 901-904.

52. Cardillo JA, Alves MR, Ambrosio LE, Porterto MB, Jose NK. Single intraoperative application versus postoperative mitomycin C eye drops in pterygium surgery. *Ophthalmology* 1995; 102 (12): 1949-1952.

53. Rubinfeld RS, Stein RM. Topical mitomycin C for pterygia: is single application appropriate? *Ophthalmic Surg. Lasers* 1997; 28 (8): 662-669.

54. Caliscan S., Orhan M., Irkec M. Intraoperative and postoperative use of mitomycin C in the treatment of primary pterygium. *Ophthalmic Surg. and Lasers* 1996; 27: 600-604.

55. Dougherty PJ, Hardten DR, Lindstrom RL. Corneoscleral melt after pterygium surgery using a single intraoperative application of mitomycin C. *Cornea* 1996; 15 (5): 537-540.

5

QUESTIONS AND ANSWERS ON PTERYGIUM MANAGEMENT

Robert L. Phillips, M.D.

INTRODUCTION

Many questions have been answered over the years regarding treatment of pterygia, yet many others remain and still others will occur in the future. Even to the present day, pterygia remain an enigma and there is no universal agreement as to the best treatment in any case. This chapter provides an attempt to answer questions which have arisen out of our historial past and a cross-section of the current conventional wisdom and treatment of this very perplexing and frustrating disease. Easy answers are not always possible, and sometimes there is no absolute dogma that exists.

1. What is the history of the pterygium?

Historical references are present that document the history of pterygia before 1000 B.C. Many unusual treatments have been employed over this period of time, including the application of powdered salt into the eye, the use of sharp hooks to remove the pterygium by avulsion, or unusual medical treatments such as mixtures of collyrium of lead, zinc, copper, iron, and even cabbage and pomegranate.

2. What are the historical theories of the etiology of pterygia?

A variety of possibilities have been put forward. Theories such as chronic irritation from wind or dust, the development of a pterygium from a pre-ceding pinguecula, and dietary deficiency such as choline have been proposed. In 1892, Fuchs published a paper putting forth a theory that the pterygium grew directly from a pinguecula. Theobald in 1877 felt that the co-contraction of the medial and lateral recti muscles produced venostasis, resulting in the growth.

3. What are current theories regarding pterygium pathogenesis?

The word "pterygium" comes from the Greek root "pterygos", which means "wing". The growth itself is observed to occur as a degenerative process at the limbus. Typically, the lesion presents at the 3 and 9 o'clock position in the area of the fissure. The nasal fissure is larger than is seen temporally, and consequently more ultraviolet light exposure occurs in that area. It is very unusual to see a lateral pterygium without the presence of a nasal pterygium, although that can occur.

Many causes may be at work in the occurrence and recurrence of pterygia, even to the molecular level. Most theories advocate the role of ultraviolet light exposure as a major predisposing factor in a primary pterygium. Other factors may be at work, such as vasoactive substances in the pathogenesis of recurrent pterygia. Other factors suggested have been blink rate, tear production, and any abnormality that causes localized drying of the cornea and the conjunctiva.

4. What is a pseudo-pterygium?

A pseudo-pterygium, or false pterygium, can occur after any inflammatory episode or chronic inflammatory disease, such as a chemical burn or some other type of trauma. In this type of pterygium, the limbus may be bridged, so that an instrument can be passed easily underneath the body of the pterygium, which is not possible with a true pterygium.

5. What pathologic changes are found in pterygia?

The histology observed in pterygia include many features that are also found in pinguecula. Electron microscopic studies of pinguecula demonstrate sub-epithelial tissue and fibers that are more prominent with elastic stain. Also demonstrated are areas of degenerated basophilic sub-epithelial fibers. Some of these fibers are sensitive to elastase, but others are not. The histologic changes found in pinguecula and pterygia are essentially identical, except that in a pterygium the superficial cornea is invaded and Bowman's layer is destroyed by fibrovascular ingrowth.

6. Are any other factors of significance?

Butras has reported in patients who underwent primary excision of pterygia the mean mast cell count per cubic millimeter was twice as high in pterygia specimens as those in age-matched controlled subjects. This elastotic and degenerative process in the conjunctiva is not well-understood, and may involve many factors, including stem-cell abnormalities resultant from a combination of factors. The proliferation of microvascular endothelial cells in tissue culture is stimulated by mast cells and may accumulate markedly at certain sites. Heparin and histamine, which are mediators of mast cells, do have vasoactive properties and could be involved in angiogenesis. It has been well-documented that Mitomycin-C does inhibit fibroblast proliferating for an extended period of time. It is also possible that Mitomycin-C might affect the interaction of mast cells with the fibroblasts.

7. How does the role of ultraviolet radiation come into play?

The ultraviolet spectrum only constitutes a small part of solar energy, but it is much more biologically active than infrared and other wavelengths that are present in greater percentages. The ultraviolet rays can cause depolymerization, molecular rearrangement, and photodecomposition, among other effects. The ozone layer in general prevents wave-lengths shorter than 2900 angstrom units from reaching the earth; however, all of that has been changing over the last several years. Those wave-lengths that are important for the formation of pterygia are in the range of 2900 to 3200 angstroms. The prevalence of pterygia seems to have a direct relationship to latitude. More equatorial latitudes have a higher incidence, but the incidence can vary even within the same latitude. The differences within latitudes might be explained in terms of air mass or cloud cover at various locations, and the quality of the air mass, such as dust content.

8. What are some of the factors involved in the recurrence of pterygia?

The geographic distribution throughout the world does not seem to affect a recurrence rate as it might affect the primary pterygium itself. Several studies have suggested that wearing of spectacle lenses with ultraviolet filters or other types of shielding devices might decrease the prevalence of a primary pterygia but would not affect the recurrence rate. Some pterygia are just simply more aggressive than others, and the younger the patient, the greater the risk of the recurrence and the greater severity of the recurrence. The stimulation from surgery may produce angiogenic factors and also accelerate fibroblastic proliferation, which is stimulated by the trauma of the surgical procedure itself.

Other factors may be important, such as alteration of the peripheral topography of the cornea, possible wetting defects, and chronic irritation produced by the surgery that may stimulate a recurrence.

One must remember that even with very excellent surgery, performed in as expert a manner as possible, recurrences are unpredictable. In Rosenthal's paper of 1953, it was stated that "You will learn from Celsus that this disease always recurs, even when you have done all in your power to cure it."

9. *Describe an outline and anatomic classification of pterygia.*

Many classification schemes exist, based on various factors. One classification system that has anatomic clarity is as follows.

Three anatomic locations of pterygia are described: cap, head, and body. The cap is the apex of the pterygium anterior to the head. Cap is defined as to represent cornea whose transparency is changed with invasion of fibroblasts from the head itself. The cap is almost always avascular, and is usually semi-opaque and flat. Sometimes, anterior to the cap may be seen some gray-white dots.

The head is considered to be the most active part of the pterygium, and the area which causes the destruction of Bowman's layer by fibrovascular ingrowth. The most anterior portion of the head may seem to be devoid of vessels, but on close inspection, usually threadlike capillaries can be identified. The head is usually elevated and can assume a variety of appearances from a fibrous and thickened appearance to a more gelatinous and fleshy, aggressive appearance. The more avascular, fibrous types of pterygia appear to recur less often, and may represent an early involutional stage.

The body of the pterygium is the area immediately posterior to the head, and much like the neck of a snake, one cannot determine where it starts and stops. As the growth advances onto the corneal surface, the conjunctiva which is adherent may begin to stretch and develop small folds. These folds may enlarge so they become redundant and overhanging, or they remain flat. There is no absolute correlation between vessels that are straight and engorged versus vessels that are more curvilinear, and the degree to which the pterygium may recur. The majority of the body is usually situated over the sclera, but in a very large pterygium it may extend onto the cornea itself. The most characteristic identifying feature of the body is the thickening of the connective tissue beneath it. The body, if extensive, may extend to the caruncle and may become very wide.

10. *Describe the relationship between a pterygium and astigmatism.*

The direction of growth of the pterygium is usually below the horizontal meridian, but can extend superiorly or inferiorly. The astigmatism produced by a pterygium may be quantitatively small, and no more than 0.5 to 1.0 diopters, but often the astigmatism is irregular and produces significant visual distortion. The axis of the astigmatism in plus cylinder is usually 90 degrees from the direction of growth of the pterygium. The pterygium produces flattening in the long axis of its growth and steepening 90 degrees away. Therefore, in plus cylinder the axis would fall between 75 and 90 degrees in the right eye. In the left eye the plus cylinder usually is more commonly between 90 and 105 degrees. As shown by topography, the astigmatism is often significantly irregular, producing symptoms of glare in difficult lighting situations.

11. *What are criteria for selection of surgical candidates in patients with a primary pterygium?*

Pterygia occurring in patients less than 40 years of age seem to represent the type of pterygia that may recur rapidly, as opposed to those occurring in older patients. If pterygium surgery is to be performed in patients less than 40 years of age, there should be some evidence that the visual acuity has decreased, the anticipation that the vision will soon be affected, or there is restriction of gaze. If the patient has a history of high ultraviolet light exposure from an outside type of occupation, extreme caution should be exercised. The decision as to whether or not to remove a pterygium for cosmetic reasons only is a matter of serious discussion between the patient and the physician, and only to be done if the patient fully understands that the recurrence might be anatomically more damaging than the original pterygium and might require further surgery. Patients can have a very simplistic idea that the growth is easy and quick to remove, and all growths by definition should be excised without any consideration for a recurrence.

12. *Which patients are candidates for a repeat surgery?*

If a recurrence occurs, and grows to the point of the previous excision and not beyond it, additional surgery may be deferred. Even though in this situation the growth has recurred in the mind of the patient, and recurrence to the previous scar is not desirable, yet if the pterygium then becomes stationary it should be observed.

If the recurrence is rapid and aggressive, and is going to grow beyond the point of the previous excision, the decision is quite different and repeat surgery is unavoidable. If vision is threatened, there is no other alternative.

13. Should initial or repeat excision be considered from a cosmetic standpoint?

This is a very difficult decision, and is made on a case-by-case basis. Thorough informed consent is necessary regarding the hazards of recurrences and multiple surgeries. There are some situations where the patient does experience discomfort with cyclical inflammation which would justify the surgery. Other individuals who work in the public arena are very concerned about the appearance of the growth from a psychosocial standpoint. The term "psychosocial" is used from the perspective that sometimes these growths are not being re-excised for purely cosmetic reasons, but for reasons that might affect one's employment and perception by the public with whom they deal.

14. What are the earliest clinical features of a pterygium?

The very earliest change that is noted in the cornea is usually just a faint haze that is composed of small, gray, dot-like opacities which can be seen at the level of Bowman's or in the subepithelial area. The pterygium itself extends onto the cornea with a variable vascular pattern and sometimes there can be some recognizable features on the head of a pterygium itself from a pre-existing pinguecula.

15. What is the clinical course of a pterygium?

Pico classifies pterygia based on their rate of growth, and this classification is useful from a clinical standpoint. The following classification is offered:

1) A stationary, or a benign pterygium will show no progression over the cornea, even over a several-year period. Fluorescein will not reveal any surface staining.

2) A progressive pterygium may advance slowly, but years may go by before it is grossly noticeable. A "malignant" or a "fleshy" pterygium may advance rapidly, with marked vasculariza-tion and congestion. The cap is usually wide and easily delineated, and punctate stain may occur in the pterygium itself or in adjacent corneal areas.

3) A cyclical type of pterygium is less ominous in terms of threatened vision, yet it can be progressive and characterized by intermittent periods of injection and chemosis with discomfort, but the progression is slower than in type 2. This type of pterygium may be treated with decongestant drops or some intermittent use of non-steroidal anti-inflammatory agents when necessary.

4) The last type is the type that will grow to a certain point and then will cease its growth at some point on the cornea. The pterygium may then contract and regress, leaving behind a scar that will be inactive, and this pterygium is called "involutional".

16. What is the relationship, if any, between a pingueculum and a pterygium?

Even though there is no certainty that a pinguecula always occurs prior to a pterygium, one cannot overlook the importance of a pinguecula in some patients. These small, fatty growths at the limbus are very common, and as the yellowish discoloration and vascularization becomes more apparent, the growth can more easily be seen without a slit-lamp. Pinguecula can certainly become symptomatic, and in some patients can precede a pterygium, although their relationship is still somewhat unclear. Almost all people over age 20, if examined carefully, will demonstrate some conjunctival thickening at the limbus representing a degenerative change of the subconjunctival connective tissue. Many pinguecula that are observed do not progress to pterygia, and many pterygia have been seen in the absence of pinguecula, so there is no absolute answer to this question.

17. What type of anesthesia should be used for pterygium surgery?

Most pterygia can be excised with subconjunctival or topical anesthesia. However, on occasion, for extensive surgery with conjunctival flaps or free grafts, a retrobulbar anesthetic may be needed. For the most complicated type of surgery, with extensive conjunctival rearrangement, where a limitation of abduction is present and dissection over the medial rectus muscle is necessary, a general anesthetic might be required.

18. What is a general technique for pterygium excision?

The type of surgery necessary will vary due to the severity of the growth. For a simple primary excision, two small buttonhole-type of incisions can be made to delineate the superior and inferior aspect of the pterygium at the limbus. The pterygium can then be avulsed using forceps or a muscle hook.

However, if the head and cap of the pterygium are extremely adherent, especially in recurrent cases, the excision may be accomplished by using a metal blade or a diamond blade, either beginning anteriorly and dissecting toward the limbus or dissecting in a reverse direction. The principal point is to try and preserve the normal topography of the cornea. Care should be exerted so that if possible a lamellar keratectomy is actually not performed, but the plane of the cornea is observed.

19. How is the diamond bur used?

I prefer a small 2.5 mm. Guibor diamond bur that is placed on a battery-operated Concept handle. The cornea portion of the excision should be polished with the diamond bur until it is entirely smooth. Sometimes microsurgical scissors might have to be used to remove small tags of tissue.

In addition, the limbal area should be polished well to remove any possible abnormal epithelial or stem cells that might be present, or abnormal fibroblasts. Obtaining a smooth limbal area and a smooth peripheral cornea is essential. One does not want to remove large amounts of tissue which creates significant wetting defects and perhaps incites a recurrence.

20. Does a bare-sclera technique have anything to recommend it?

Bare-sclera is still a commonly-used technique in pterygium surgery. In my opinion, a bare-sclera technique should never be used when Mitomycin is employed due to the possibility of poor healing.

Many surgeons feel that a bare-sclera will pro-

duce a successful operation if reasonably healthy conjunctiva is approximated at the edge of the scleral resection. Subconjunctival scar tissue should be carefully dissected, and the use of cautery should be minimal. Limbal ischemia can always be created with the surgery, and can produce peripheral ulceration.

The literature contains conflicting reports as to the success of bare-sclera technique, as it is difficult to compare one procedure with another due to a lack of uniformity and various lengths of followup.

Some authors have indicated that a bare-sclera technique allows a trans-limbal migration of the corneal epithelium and anchoring of the conjunctival epithelium to the bare sclera at its point of contact with the corneal epithelium. Then a new extracorneal pterygium begins to develop at the apex of this extracorneal epithelium and moves toward the limbus within a few weeks. The only dogmatic statement that can be made about a bare-sclera technique is that one should never use Mitomycin with this particular technique due to the extreme risk of persistent conjunctival and scleral ulceration. Restoring the normal anatomy by the use of conjunctival flaps or grafts seems more physiologic to some authors, but there is no doubt that bare-sclera technique does work.

21. Should a lamellar keratectomy be used?

If used, a lamellar keratectomy should be very, very superficial, only to remove the subepithelial fibrosis and scar tissue that is irregular and would produce an uneven surface. Dissection must be as smooth as possible, and must not be carried any deeper than is absolutely necessary to remove the growth and its attachments to the cornea. Remember, the goal is not to reach clear cornea, but simply to preserve the normal peripheral topography and just separate the pterygium from the cornea itself. In severe pterygia, Bowman's layer has already been destroyed and some anterior corneal lamella may have been destroyed, as well. A smooth, superficial dissection is to be preferred over a deep, irregular dissection. Cautery may be used for hemostasis, but care must be taken not to avoid significant limbal ischemia by too-aggressive cauterization.

22. How should free conjunctival grafts be harvested?

The superior bulbar conjunctiva provides the easiest access. A limbal stay suture should be placed and the globe rotated inferiorly. A subconjunctival anesthesia may be given to dissect the conjunctiva from the underlying Tenon's. This area is easily approachable, and the excision of the conjunctival graft can be begun superiorly, much as if one were going to begin a Gundersen conjunctival flap. A very large piece of conjunctiva may be taken and the conjunctival dissection can be carried down to the limbus. The insertion of the superior rectus muscle must not be left exposed, and the principle is not to leave two raw surfaces opposing each other, to avoid a symblepharon. One can slide the dissected conjunctiva down from its location superiorly to cover the resected area, and then suturing can be begun. Care must be taken not to invert this thin tissue, as it is very easy to do so.

23. What factors are to be considered in the use of a cautery?

Many types of cautery can be used, but normally a wet field (bipolar) cautery would be used, or perhaps an intraocular pencil cautery. The idea is to provide hemostasis, but to minimize any tissue damage which might stimulate regrowth of sub conjunctival scar tissue. A heavy and aggressive use of cautery could produce a more pronounced scar, or, in extreme circumstances, could even precipitate limbal ischemia.

24. In general terms, what is the role of the use of beta-irradiation?

Beta-irradiation is an adjunctive measure that can be used either for aggressive primary or recurrent pterygia. The effect of the radiation is to produce ionization changes in the nucleus and cytoplasm of the cells, and the cells that are most sensitive to the radiation are the endothelium of newly-developing capillaries. An endarteritis is produced in these capillaries, and fibroblast proliferation is prevented. One can put on an initial amount of radiation at the time of surgery, and then perhaps a second amount a week later, when the newly-developing capillaries are beginning to form. The exact use of the beta-irradiation is not standardized in terms of dose or time of application, but many papers consistently report lower recurrence rates with its use.

25. How is Thio-tepa used?

Thio-tepa is triethylene thiophosphoramide. The use of Thio-tepa or nitrogen mustard has been advocated for several years, and was initially reported by Meachum in 1952 in the *American Journal of Ophthalmology*. This drug is a radiomimetic agent that, like beta-irradiation, obliterates newly-forming capillaries at the surgical site and inhibits the endothelium from growing. Its use is effective and well-documented. Concentrations described have been from 1:1,000 or 1:2,000, four to six times per day for 6 to 8 weeks after surgery. One must be cautious in those patients who manifest allergy to the drug, and particularly cautious of darker-skinned patients. Thio-tepa can create depigmentation on the lids if it overflows onto the face, as melanocytes are very sensitive to this medication. Patients with darker skin, therefore, must be warned about this complication.

26. What role do steroids play?

Steroid drops are used with virtually all techniques to control inflammation after surgery. The inhibition of inflammation produced by steroids may prevent vascularization and rapid re-growth of the pterygium in some patients. The steroids may be started before the epithelium has healed, as long as the patient is compliant and will return for post-operative visits on schedule. The dosage can be adjusted based on the inflammatory response in each patient.

27. What are some of the factors in recurrent pterygia?

Recurrences occur no matter what precautions one takes, either medical or surgical. The recurrence rate is highly individual, and is probably multifactorial. Patients under age 40, with large, engorged vessels on the pterygia, tend to have a high recurrence rate, especially those with a history of significant ultraviolet light exposure. The surgery itself can also be a precipitating event, as each individual has a different inflammatory response. Leaving behind an irregular corneal surface is a known risk factor, and also leaving behind irregular soft tissue elevations over the sclera or at the limbus. The limbal area needs to be polished carefully to rid the area of all abnormal epithelial cells that could have a potential to produce scar tissue and recurrence. Stem cell abnormalities at the limbus undoubtedly play a role in this disease and its recurrence, and that area continues to be defined.

28. *What is the role of free conjunctival grafts?*

Free conjunctival grafts have been used for many years. Placement of a graft or a flap insures a more proper wound healing by returning the surface of the globe to its normal presurgical state. Kenyon's paper in 1985 in *Ophthalmology* describes a technique used in conjunctival grafts from the superior bulbar conjunctiva.

29. *Can buccal mucosal grafts still be used?*

Yes, mucosal grafts have been used for many years, and require the use of a mucotome to obtain a thickness of approximately .1 to .2 mm. The mucosa can shred if it is too thin, and care must be employed. The same cosmetic result is not obtainable with mucosa as can be obtained with conjunctiva, but when conjunctiva is not available, this modality can be used. The mucosa is obtained from the lower lip after making the lip turgid with the injection of saline.

30. *What is the rationale for amnion grafts?*

The biologic process of wound healing produces fibrosis, but does not always result in the complete restoration of the function of the tissue. If the epithelial basement membrane is damaged, an amnion graft which contains a thick basement membrane and an avascular, extracellular matrix will allow healing without scarring. Amnion contains protease inhibitors and other factors which may allow the establishment of a more normal phenotype for cells. Some anti-angiogenic factors may also be present.

31. *How can amniotic membrane be obtained?*

Preserved amniotic membrane can be harvested from a placenta obtained from a Cesarean section

delivery. The amnion is separated from the chorion, and must be prepared in specific fashion based on nitrocellulose filter paper and frozen. This technique is described in the chapter by Dr. Scheffer Tseng. Dr. Tseng has developed a specific protocol for preparation of amnion. IRB approval is probably not needed, as this is a standard technique, but each institution may be somewhat different. It is much easier to use the amnion when it has been pre-prepared, as the technique for its preparation is very labor-intensive. Currently amnion is available from Bio-Tissue, Inc., in South Miami, as well as from Tissue Banks International. Their addresses are as follows:

	Address	*Phone Number*
BIO-Tissue, Inc.	6601 S.W. 80th Street, Suite #200B South Miami, Florida 33143	(305) 669-1318
Tissue Banks, International	815 Park Avenue Baltimore, Maryland 21201-4848	(410) 752-3800

32. *Are there any other uses for amnion?*

More and more uses for amniotic membrane are being defined. It is used for the surface reconstruction of the conjunctiva and cornea in a variety of situations, including chemical or thermal trauma, pemphigoid, symblepharon, Stevens-Johnson, and contact lens-induced stem cell keratopathy. Amnion is obviously also useful in conjunctival reconstruction in severe recurrent pterygia.

33. *When should a lamellar keratoplasty be employed?*

Most surgeons feel that a keratoplasty should be reserved for the most severe recurrences that cannot be managed in any other way. The procedure is more technically demanding, but when carefully performed, a keratoplasty offers an excellent chance to prevent any further recurrences.

34. *What is a technique for lamellar keratoplasty for recurrent pterygia?*

I have used Poirier's technique on a number of

cases and have found it to be effective and easy to teach to our residents. An 8 mm., .3 mm. thickness lamellar corneal button is employed. It can be free-hand-dissected from a whole globe, or a microkeratome can be used. The pterygium is excised in a normal manner. An 8 mm. trephine is used to make a mark to facilitate the lamellar dissection on the host; 3 mm. is onto the corneal surface and approximately 5 mm. onto the scleral surface. A lamellar bed is prepared to accept the .3 mm. lamellar tissue. As in most extensive recurrent pterygia, it is essential to isolate the medial rectus so its insertion can be identified and damage can be avoided. The .3 mm. lamellar button is placed into the pre-prepared lamellar bed and sutured with interrupted 10-0 Ethilon.

35. What are the most common difficulties in lamellar keratoplasty?

The dissection must be done with great caution to avoid perforation, especially if there is previous thinning of the tissues. The medial rectus can be inadvertently damaged, so its identification and the placement of a suture beneath it is always helpful. The exact position of the trephine can be modified somewhat, depending upon the involvement of the pupillary space and scar tissue, but again, caution must be employed for this portion of the procedure.

36. Do pterygia recur with a lamellar keratoplasty?

In my experience, I have thus far never had a recurrent pterygium when a lamellar keratoplasty was used. One can often see vessels growing in the lamellar bed, but once they reach a certain point they apparently lose their nutritional support, and they begin to fragment and break up. Poirier feels that there is a graft-host interface barrier to regrowth of the pterygium.

37. When was Mitomycin first used?

Kunitomo and Mori in Japan first reported the usefulness of the postoperative instillation of Mitomycin. In their original work, .4 mg/cc was used three times per day for 1 to 2 weeks. The medication was widely used in Japan, and some investigators even used a strength of 1.0 mg/cc. Initial complications observed included scleral ulceration, fail-

ure to re-epithelialize of either the cornea or conjunctiva, iridocyclitis and secondary glaucoma. Tseng, Wilson, and Foster reported in 1988 a study comparing 1.0 mg/cc of Mitomycin and another group using .4 mg/cc. The 1.0 mg/cc created significant complications, and those complications were minimized by using then .4 mg/cc.

38. What is the current thinking on the proper dose of Mitomycin?

The pharmacokinetics of this drug are still being investigated, and there currently are no absolutes. In 1989, Hayasaka and colleagues reported data that suggested .2 mg/cc of the Mitomycin could be considered safe and effective in the treatment of recurrent pterygia. Hayasaka used the medication twice daily for five days. At the present time, most pterygia surgeons feel that a topical application of Mitomycin onto the surgical site as a single application, followed by copious irrigation, is much safer than the use of Mitomycin ad a postoperative drop.

39. What is the pharmacology of Mitomycin?

Mitomycin is manufactured in the United States by Bristol Laboratories under the trade name Mutamycin. The drug is an antibiotic that is isolated from the broth of Streptomyces caespitosus, which is known to have anti-tumor activity. Mitomycin selectively inhibits the synthesis of DNA and cellular RNA and protein synthesis are also suppressed. Used systemically in the treatment of adenocarcinoma of the stomach or pancreas, it does have bone marrow toxicity, but when used topically no systemic adverse reactions have been reported.

40. How is Mitomycin formulated?

To formulate Mitomycin ophthalmic solution in a strength of 0.4 mg/mL, the procedure is as follows:
1) dissolve the contents of one vial of Mitomycin (Mutamycin) which is 5 mg., in 12.5 milliliters of sterile water without preservatives;
2) place the contents in a 2 ounce sterile dropper bottle;
3) final product equals 0.4 mg/mL.

The expiration date is approximately 14 days,

and chemotherapeutic precautions should be observed in the compounding of this product, such as the use of a laminar flow hood. If the sterile water amount is increased to 25.0 mL, a concentration of .2 mg/mL would be achieved.

41. How should Mitomycin be applied in the operating room?

The most effective way to apply this drug during pterygium surgery has not yet been completely determined. A Weck cell sponge may be used to apply the drug directly to the resected area. Cotton pledgets can also be used to apply the drug much as is used in glaucoma filtration surgery. I currently apply the Mitomycin in a strength of 0.2 mg/mL with a Weck cell sponge for approximately two minutes. That is followed by irrigation with a copious amount of balanced salt solution.

42. Why is Mitomycin not used as a postoperative drop?

One must remember that Mitomycin is a very powerful and very dangerous drug, but when used appropriately, risks are usually controllable to a reasonable degree. Direct application to the resected scleral bed is effective in preventing recurrence of subcon-junctival fibrosis and extension of these fibroblasts onto the corneal surface. It is not used as a postoperative drop by most surgeons because in a non-compliant patient, the control of its use is not possible. This drug is potentially too dangerous to allow the patient to use it in a drop form after surgery for fear of its misuse.

43. Can complications occur with a single intraoperative application?

Unfortunately, the answer to this question is yes. Cases of a rupture of the globe after seemingly minor trauma have occurred after a single application in the operating room. For this reason it must be carefully explained to patients that the pharmacokinetics of this drug are still not completely understood, and even with a single application in the operating room, complications such as scleral or conjunctival ulceration can occur. This drug is FDA approved in the United States for use in adenocarcinomas of the stomach and pancreas. Its use in pterygium surgery is an off-label use, and this must be explained in detail to the patient. Use of Mitomycin should be included on the operative permit.

44. What should I look for at the slit-lamp in terms of a complication from Mitomycin?

One must observe the conjunctiva and the cornea in a meticulous fashion for a non-healing epithelial defect, conjunctival wound separation, and persistent conjunctival or corneal defects that could lead to ulceration and non-healing. One can observe a very whitened appearance of the eye in the area of the pterygium excision and Mitomycin application, as newly-forming capillaries do not tend to populate the area very rapidly. Staining is often necessary to recognize the presence of conjunctival epithelium.

45. Can a bare sclera technique be used in combination with Mitomycin?

Absolutely not. If there is anything that is absolutely axiomatic in this chapter, it would be that bare sclera should never be used in conjunction with Mitomycin.

Many surgeons do use a bare sclera technique with success, but in my opinion it is definitely not to be recommended with the concomitant use of such a powerful drug as Mitomycin. The risk of scleral or corneal ulceration is greatly enhanced when the sclera is not completely closed and Mitomycin has been applied.

46. Should the Weck cell sponge or cotton pledget touch the conjunctival edge when applied?

It is virtually impossible to avoid application of Mitomycin to the conjunctival edge, no matter how carefully one tries. Theoretically one would want the edge to possess some fibroblastic activity so that healing can occur with a conjunctival flap or free graft. Based on many cases from a large number of investigators, the fact that the edge of the conjunctiva happens to touch the Weck cell sponge did not seem to interfere with healing in most cases. One must remember that there is individual variation from patient to patient.

47. Can a surgeon control the level of Mitomycin-C delivered?

Lee and Heuer are glaucoma specialists who have made some comments and suggestions to try and effect a better control of the drug delivery. No matter how we can control the delivery, long-term effects of the drug cannot be predicted with absolute certainty. Before one begins using Mitomycin, the surgeon needs to be very familiar with everything that is known about its pharmacokinetics and its complications. Here are some of the issues that Lee and Heuer suggest should be considered:

1. The decision whether or not to use an antimetabolite, and if so, which antimetabolite?
2. The concentration of Mitomycin-C to be used.
3. How should it be applied - with a cotton pledget, a Weck cell sponge, or some other method?
4. The duration of treatment.
5. The point during the procedure at which the Mitomycin is applied.
6. How do we handle the application of the drug to Tenon's or to the conjunctival edge, or to the area of resection itself.

48. Is Mitomycin used in all surgical pterygia cases?

No; in primary pterygia that appear not to be very aggressive, I think a standard surgical technique can be employed.

49. In what cases is Mitomycin recommended?

Some of these decisions are individual judgements made by the individual surgeon. I tend to use the drug in very aggressive primary pterygia, especially in young patients, or in pterygia involving multiple recurrences.

50. What are factors to be considered in the choice of type of material used to apply the Mitomycin?

The best delivery system has probably not been attained at present. One can section small pieces of Weck cell sponges or cotton, or one can use an instrument wipe to apply the Mitomycin. Some sponge-like materials may release more Mitomycin than others. The goal is to apply the drug directly to the area where you want it, and not have it release into other areas of the globe. Based on my experience, I believe that suitable concentrations of the drug can be obtained by using Weck cell sponges or cotton pledgets, or Muracel sponges placed directly beneath the conjunctiva, and draping the conjunctiva over these materials. The timing must be cautious, employing either two or three minutes, and then irrigation of copious amounts of balanced salt solution is required.

51. Are there any absolute contraindications to Mitomycin use?

Rubenfeld and others feel that there are some definite contraindications to Mitomycin use. There is some consensus that Mitomycin is probably contraindicated in patients who have the following diseases: keratitis sicca, neurotrophic disease, patients with inadequate blink or lagophthalmos, and patients in general who are in poor health and may manifest evidence of connective tissue disorders such as rheumatoid arthritis. These patients tend in general to heal poorly, with poor fibroblastic activity, so sometimes the addition of Mitomycin in this scenario can be disastrous.

52. Do you do anything differently in terms of Mitomycin and an informed surgical consent form?

I do use a standard consent form, because the use of Mitomycin in glaucoma surgery and pterygium surgery, and more recently, in the use of squamous cell carcinomas is well-documented and established, supported by many papers from many investigators. But even with all of this clinical evidence of its effectiveness, written information should be placed in the patient's chart that one has explained the possible risks of this drug, the fact that the use of this drug in this type of surgery is an off-label use, and a full explanation has been given regarding its risks and benefits. This information could be incorporated into a consent form, but at the least it certainly should be written into the chart in an admission note or office visit that all of this information has been fully explained.

53. Is there any evidence that Mitomycin could have an effect on the graft/host junction in a keratoplasty procedure?

Yes, there is a case reported in the *Archives of Ophthalmology* in 1995 by a group from Houston, Texas. The patient had had a keratoplasty following an alkali burn, and later required a trabeculectomy where Mitomycin was required. Subsequent to the filtration procedure, the filtering bleb became ischemic, the limbus thinned, and the graft/host interface dehisced, which resulted in prolapse and incarceration. Other factors may have been involved here, but there is the suggestion that Mitomycin could have affected the healing at the graft/host interface.

54. What would be a comparison of the use of Mitomycin-C in conjunctival autografts and excision of pterygia?

Published studies indicate that these two procedures may be considered essentially equal in effectiveness. As has been previously stated, there are many individual factors in recurrence of pterygium even to the molecular level, and even with all the studies published thus far it is difficult to be dogmatic. Recurrence rates can be defined differently in different studies, which can affect published results.

55. Is beta-irradiation effective?

Beta-irradiation is generally accepted to be an effective method of reduction of the rate of recurrence of pterygia. The exact dose to be used and the timing of delivery varies among surgeons. There is no absolute uniformity. Beta rays are electrons that cause ionization of atoms of biologic tissues through which they pass. As they pass through the tissues and cause this ionization, electrons are ejected from the atoms to the cells, and this causes an alteration in the biochemistry of the cells. The goal, as in other modalities, is to cause inhibition of the growth of fibroblasts and blood vessels in the subconjunctival connective tissue stage without producing an overdose. Beta-irradiation penetrates very superficially. The cornea, sclera, uvea, retina and ciliary body are relatively radioresistant to a high degree. The germinal equatorial cells in the lens are very sensitive. Beta-irradiation does not appear to be useful for pterygia that are already established, and it has its most beneficial effect on rapidly-growing immature tissue which occurs after surgery.

56. How do you calibrate a strontium-90 applicator?

Strontium-90 applicators (beta-irradiation) must continue to be calibrated, probably at about six month intervals. Two applicators may be of identical size, of the same type, and even have the same amount of radioactive material. Yet these applicators may vary in total energy output, surface dose rates, and depth dose. Depth dose refers to a falloff of the surface dose at succeeding levels of penetration. Surface output only refers to the quantity of emitted electrons, and says nothing about their energy or their penetrating power. Depth dose information is obviously important to consider the possibility of cataract formation.

57. What is strontium-90?

Isotope strontium-90 emits beta-irradiation, and the strontium-90 has a half-life of 28 years. The strontium-90 is a fission product, and decays to Yttrium-90 with a half-life of 64 hours, and there is no Gamma emission. The strength of the applicator varies, and it should be re-calibrated approximately every six months, as the amount of emission varies with time. A great advantage of the beta applicator is its depth-dose pattern. The beta rays have their maximum effect on the surface 2 mm. of tissue, where the effect is needed the most.

58. How should beta-irradiation be applied?

There is no standard protocol for the application of beta-irradiation, and differences occur among surgeons. The consensus seems to be that no more than about 2000 rads of total irradiation needs to be applied. This may be split such that 1000 rads are applied at the time of surgery and a week later an additional 1000 are applied. However, some surgeons apply a total dose of between 1000 and 2000 at the time of the initial surgery and none beyond that date. No consensus exists on the total dosage, the optimum time of delivery, and the need for fractionation of the delivery.

59. Can a cataract be induced by beta-irradiation?

It is well-documented and accepted that cataract changes can be induced by beta-irradiation due to penetration of the rays to the equatorial area of the lens. Even in patients who do not develop a clinical cataract, oftentimes with wide dilation one can see minute, dot-like opacities near the periphery of the lens that presumably come from the radiation itself. Ionizing radiation initially injures the equatorial cells of the lens epithelium, and subsequent changes appear in lens fibers, particularly in the posterior capsular region.

In order to produce a visually significant cataract in the pupillary space, a very large dose is required, something in the range of 8000-10,000 rads. This far exceeds the normal dose that is applied in pterygium surgery. There are many variables involved, so the exact type of cataract being produced cannot be predicted in every patient, but the development of a clinically significant cataract is very unusual.

60. What are some of the complications of treatment with strontium-90?

Complications that have been reported are thinning of the sclera, scleral or corneal ulceration, or even perforation. In most cases, these complications are related to a total dose.

61. What are some basic safety precautions using a strontium-90 applicator?

If not handled properly, unnecessary radiation can expose the skin to damage. One should never touch the tip of the applicator, and it should only be manipulated by the handle provided. By holding the shielded handle, the user will not be exposed significantly. The unshielded end of the instrument should never be pointed at any individual and the manufacturer-supplied handling tongs should be used for the placement and removal of the beam collimating mass on the applicator tip. The applicator should be stored in an individual storage case which is clearly identified. A radiation safety officer should have overall control of the storage and proper calibration of the instrument. When cleaning the applicator tip, the shielding handle should be used and the tip may be wiped across a cotton swab, sponge, or gauze with a sterilizing agent on a flat surface. The applicator tip should never be touched by the fingers.

62. Is a license necessary to use beta-irradiation?

In the United States, a license must be obtained from the Nuclear Regulatory Commission to use the beta-irradiation device, and personal dosimeters should be used when handling the applicator. Evidence of training in the use of a beta-irradiation applicator must be provided, and obtaining the license can be a lengthy process. Sometimes an individual can sign on to another person's application that has already been received, with the proper endorsement.

63. What role does an Argon laser play in recurrent pterygia?

Argon blue-green lasers are not effective in treating primary pterygia, but may be successful in some early recurrences. Cases best suited for laser therapy are those where the excision has been optimum and the corneal surface is smooth. If vascularization is occurring due to an irregular surface, due to probable surface hypoxia, the laser may not be effective.

64. When should laser therapy be considered?

If one is a proponent of laser therapy, the patient should be carefully observed on a weekly basis for approximately 8 to 10 weeks. If neovascular tufts are observed, the laser should be applied to these immature vessels and should not be delayed into the vessels are established and onto the corneal surface. The conjunctiva should not be burned in order to avoid further fibrosis and inflammation. Only the vessels themselves should be closed, and no other effect is desired.

65. What is the technique of Argon laser use in recurrent pterygia?

The period of observation is very important in the use of laser, and the patient should be observed on a weekly basis until the eye is quiet. The new vessel fronds should be treated at intervals approximately one to two weeks apart, and the maximum number of applications will usually average between 2 and 4. Time here is very important, and that is why careful observation is necessary, to treat these vessels at their most vulnerable stage. The interval between treatments might be one to two weeks, or it could be as long as six weeks.

66. *What laser power settings should be used?*

The correct power may vary somewhat from patient to patient, but the power in general should be enough to ablate the vessel but not thermally burn the conjunctiva. Usually a 50 micron spot size, interval of 0.1 seconds, and a power of 0.2 to 0.3 watts is adequate. The laser should be placed in three to four parallel rows, equidistant to each other and parallel to the limbus.

66. *What type of anesthesia is needed in Argon laser application?*

Topical anesthesia in the average patient usually is sufficient. On occasions, there may be a patient who is unusually sensitive, who may require subconjunctival anesthesia, although sometimes this will distort the vascular pattern. On occasions, retrobulbar anesthesia might be needed, but the necessity for this type of anesthesia is uncommon.

67. *What does the future hold?*

Undoubtedly, many drugs in the future will be developed that may have application to pterygium surgery. The delivery mechanisms of these drugs continue to be investigated so that more precise drugs can be delivered to a given site. Bioadhesive polymers or biodegradable polymers that deliver a drug to an eye on a controlled and sustained basis will be a subject of continued research. Continued efforts will be made to determine the optimum drug dose and the delivery method to avoid significant complications. The use of laser to remove pterygia in future applications and amnion membranes hold promise for the future.

68. *What is your routine surgical technique for the use of amnion?*

The amnion can be used as a single layer, or can be folded. Dr. Scheffer C.G. Tseng recommends that when it is folded, the two stromal sides should face each other while keeping the basement membrane side on the external portion. Folding can be used to increase the thickness of the tissue where there has been a previous lamellar keratectomy and there is some peripheral corneal thinning. The folding is also useful when there is restriction of motility, because the lower layer serves in a fashion to simulate a new muscle sheath that prevents fibrous tissue from forming and re-restriction of the muscle. Adjacent conjunctival autografts can also be used near the strip to aid in re-epithelialization.

69. *How far should the amnion extend?*

The amnion could extend no further than the limbus, but it is often useful to allow an overlapping of the amnion out onto the corneal surface that covers the area occupied by the defect created when the head of the pterygium is removed. The objection of fashioning the membrane to cover the corneal portion of the dissection would be to allow the surrounding epithelium to expand to cover the defect, and according to Dr. Tseng, to present the "corneal stroma being denuded and exposed to tear PMN's", as the latter are a key source of recurrence.

70. *Can Mitomycin-C be used with a conjunctival graft?*

I think this issue is not yet decided at the present time, and I would urge extreme caution in using conjunctival grafts with Mitomycin. There may be certain cases that might be successful, and others that could be disastrous. At the present time I do not believe this issue has been studied well enough to state with confidence that conjunctiva could be used with Mitomycin. It has recently been reported, however, that intraoperative Mitomycin and amnion membrane transplants have been used in some cicatricial cases. This issue needs to be studied further.

REFERENCES

1. Aswad MI, Baum J. Optimal time for postoperative irradiation of pterygia. *Ophthalmology* 94:1450-1451, 1987.

2. Azuara-Blanco A, Pillai CT, Dua HS. Amniotic membrane transplantation for ocular surface reconstruction. Br J Ophthalmol 1999; 83: 399-402.

3. Butrus SI, Ashraf MF, Laby DM, Rabinowitz, AI, Tabbara SO, and Hidayat, AA. Increased numbers of Mast cells in pterygia. *AJO* 119:236-237, 1995.

4. Campbell OR, Amendola, BE, Brady LW: Recurrent pterygia: results of postoperative treatment with Sr-90 applicators. *Radiology* 1990: 174, 565-566.

5. Chen PP, Ariyasu RG, Kaza V, LaBree LD, McDonald PJ. A randomized trial comparing mitomycin-C and conjunctival autograft after excision of primary pterygium. *AJO* 120-2; 151-160, 1995.

6 Dougherty, Hardten, Lindstrom. Corneoscleral melt after pterygium surgery using a single intraoperative application of Mitomycin-C". *Cornea* 15: 537-542, 1996.

7. Dushku N, Reid TW. Immunohistochemical evidence that human pterygia originate from an invasion of vimentin-expressing altered limbal epithelial basal cells. *Current Eye Research* 473-481, 1994.

8 . Dushku N, Reid TW. P53 expression in altered limbal basal cells of pingueculae, pterygia, and limbal tumors. *Current Eye Research* 1179-1192, 1997.

9. Haik GM, Ellis GS, Nowell JF. The management of pterygia with special reference to surgery combined with beta irradiation. *Tr Am Acad Ophth & Otol* 776-784, Nov-Dec 1982.

10. Hayasaka S, Noda S, Yamamoto Y, Setogawa T. Postoperative instillation of low-dose mitomycin C in the treatment of primary pterygium. *Am J Ophthalmol* 106: 715-718, 1988.

11. Hayasaka S, Noda S, Yamamota Y, et. al. Postoperative instillation of Mitomycin C in the treatment of recurrent pterygium. *Ophthalmic Surgery* 20, 580-583, 1989.

12. Hayasaka S, Noda S, Yamamoto Y Setogawa T. Postoperative instillation of mitomycin C in the treatment of recurrent pterygium. <u>Ophthalmic Surg</u> 20: 580-583, 1989.

13. Hayasaka S, Noda S, Yamamoto Y, Setogawa T. Reply to Singh G: Postoperative instillation of low-dose mitomycin C in the treatment of primary pterygium [correspondence]. *Am J Ophthalmol* 107: 571, 1989.

14. Hirst LW, Sebban A, Chant D. Pterygium recurrence time. *Ophthalmol* 100; 755-758, 1994.

15. Kenyon KR, Wagoner MD, Hettinger ME. Conjunctival autograft transplantation for advanced and recurrent pterygium. *Ophthalmology* 92: 461-70, 1985.

16. Kim JC, Tseng SCG. Transplantation of presumed human amniotic membrane for surface of reconstruction in severely damaged rabbit corneas. *Invest Ophthalmol Vis Sci* 34(S): 1366, 1993.

17. Kunitomo N, Mori S. Studies on the pterygium, 4: a treatment of the pterygium by mitomycin C instillation. *Acta Soc Ophthalmol Jpn* 67; 601-607, 1963.

18. Kwok LS, Coroneo MT. A model for pterygium formation. *Cornea* 13(3): 219-224, 1994.

19. Lam DSC, Wong AKK, Fan DSP et al. Intraoperative mitomycin C to prevent recurrence of pterygium after excision: A 30-month follow-up study. *Ophthalmology* 105, 901-905, 1998.

20. Laughrea PA, Arentsen JJ. Lamellar keratoplasty in the management of recurrent pterygium. *Ophthalmic Surgery* 17, 106-108, 1986.

21. MacKenzie FD, Hirst LW; Battistutta D, Green A. Risk analysis in the development of pterygia. *Ophthalmology* 99: 1056-1061, 1992.

22. Mahar PS, Nwokora GE. Role of mitomycin C in pterygium surgery. *Br J Ophthalmol* 77, 433-435, 1993.

23. Manning CA, Kloess PM, Diaz MD, Yee RW. Intraoperative Mitomycin in primary pterygium excision: A prospective, randomized trial. *Ophthalmology* 104, 844-848, 1997.

24. Pico G. Pterygium - current concept of etiology and management. From King JH, McTigue JWA (eds): *The Cornea World Congress*, Butterworth, Washington, D.C.: 280-291, 1965.

25. Pires RTF, Tseng SCG, Prabhasawat P, Puangsricharern V, Maskin SL, Kim JC, and Tan DTH. Amniotic membrane transplantation for symptomatic bullous keratopathy. *Arch Ophthalmol* 117: 1291-1297, 1999.

26. Poirier RH, Fish JR. Lamellar keratoplasty for recurrent pterygium. *Ophthalmic Surgery* 7, 38-41, 1976.

27. Rosenthal G, Shoham A, Lifshitz T, Biedner B, Yassur Y. The use of mitomycin in pterygium surgery. *Ann Ophthalmol* 25; 427-428, 1993.

28. Rubenfeld, RS, Pfister RR, Stein RM, et. al. Serious complications of topical Mitomycin-C after pterygium surgery. *Ophthalmology* 95:, 1647-1654, 1992.

29. Singh G, Wilson MR, Foster CS. Mitomycin eye drops as treatment for pterygium. *Ophthalmology* 95: 813-821, 1988.

30. Singh G, Wilson MR, Foster CS. Long-term follow-up study of mitomycin eye drops as adjunctive treatment for pterygia and its comparison with conhjunctival autograft transplantation. *Cornea* 9; 331-334, 1990.

31. Skuta, Beeson et. al. Intraoperative Mitomycin versus postoperative 5-FU in high-risk glaucoma filtering surgery. *Ophthalmology* 99, 438-444, 1992.

32. Stark T, Kenyon KR, Serrano F. Conjunctival autograft for primary and recurrent pterygia: surgical technique and problem management. *Cornea* 10; 196-202, 1991.

33. Sugar A. Who should receive Mitomycin-C after pterygium surgery? *Ophthalmology* 99,1645-1646, 1992.

34. Threlfall TJ, English, DR. Sun exposure and pterygium of the eye: a dose-response curve. *AJO* 128: 280-287, 1999.

35. U.S. Nuclear Regulatory Commission, Office of Nuclear Safety and Safeguards, Washington, D.C. *NRC Information Notice* No. 90-58 - Improper handling of ophthalmic strontium-90 beta radiation applicators. September 11, 1990.

36. Wong VA, Law FCH. Use of Mitomycin C with conjunctival autograft in pterygium surgery in Asian-Canadians. *Ophthalmology* 106; 1512-1515, 1999.